Lecture Notes on Epidemiology and Public Health Medicine

RICHARD FARMER
MB PhD FFPHM MRGCP
Professor of Community Medicine,
Charing Cross and Westminster Medical School,
University of London

DAVID MILLER
MD FRCP FFPHM
Professor of Community Medicine,
St Mary's Hospital Medical School,
Imperial College of Science, Technology
and Medicine, University of London

THIRD EDITION

OXFORD

BLACKWELL SCIENTIFIC PUBLICATIONS

LONDON EDINBURGH BOSTON

MELBOURNE PARIS BERLIN VIENNA

© 1977, 1983, 1991 by
Blackwell Scientific Publications
Editorial Offices:
Osney Mead, Oxford OX2 0EL
25 John Street, London WC1N 2BL
23 Ainslie Place, Edinburgh EH3 6AJ
3 Cambridge Center, Cambridge
  Massachusetts 02142, USA
54 University Street, Carlton
  Victoria 3053, Australia

Other Editorial Offices:
Arnette SA
2, rue Casimir-Delavigne
75006 Paris
France

Blackwell Wissenschaft
Meinekestrasse 4
D-1000 Berlin 15
Germany

Blackwell MZV
Feldgasse 13
A-1238 Wien
Austria

First published in 1977 under the title
Lecture Notes on Epidemiology and
Community Medicine
Second edition 1983
Reprinted 1984, 1985, 1986,
  1987 (twice), 1988
Third edition 1991

Set by Times Graphics, Singapore
Printed and bound in Great Britain by
Billing and Sons Ltd, Worcester

DISTRIBUTORS

Marston Book Services Ltd
PO Box 87
Oxford OX2 0DT
(*Orders*: Tel: 0865-791155
        Fax: 0865-791927
        Telex: 837515)

USA
Mosby-Year Book, Inc.
11830 Westline Industrial Drive
St Louis, Missouri 63146
(*Orders*: Tel: (800) 633-6699)

Canada
Mosby-Year Book, Inc.
5240 Finch Avenue East
Scarborough, Ontario
(*Orders*: Tel: (416) 298-1588)

Australia
Blackwell Scientific Publications
(Australia) Pty Ltd
54 University Street
Carlton, Victoria 3053
(*Orders*: Tel: (03) 347-0300)

British Library
Cataloguing in Publication Data

Farmer, R.D.T.
  Lecture notes on epidemiology and public
  health medicine. — 3rd. ed.
  1. Community medicine. Epidemiological
  methods
  I. Title II. Miller, D.L. (David
  Louis) III. Farmer, R.D.T.
  Lecture notes on epidemiology and
  community medicine
  362.10425

ISBN 0-632-02412-7

Lecture Notes on Epidemiology and Public Health Medicine

Contents

Preface

In order to safeguard and improve the health of society, whatever its stage of development, it is essential to understand why diseases arise. To do this it is necessary to study the distribution and natural history of disease in populations, so that societies can devise and plan preventive programmes and services for the sick.

The discipline of public health medicine is concerned with these aspects of medical practice. It rarely involves direct therapeutic intervention with patients. Essentially the subject is concerned with raising the level of health of groups of people and with meeting their collective ambitions for a better quality of life.

In the text, the pronoun he is used to refer to doctors and patients. This is not intended to imply that all doctors and patients are male, and we hope that the reader is not offended by what has been adopted as an economical linguistic convention.

Acknowledgement
We are greatly indebted to Dr Carl Burns for his assistance in the production of this edition.

List of Abbreviations Used

AHA	Area Health Authority
CDSC	Communicable Disease Surveillance Centre
CRS	Congenital Rubella Syndrome
DHA	District Health Authority
DIS	District Information System
DTP	Diphtheria Tetanus Pertussis
FPC	Family Practitioner Committee
GHS	General Household Survey
HAA	Hospital Activity Analysis
HIPE	Hospital In-Patient Enquiry
HNIG	Human Normal Immunoglobin
HSE	Health and Safety Executive
ICD	International Classification of Diseases
IHD	Ischaemic Heart Disease
LDLC	Low Density Lipoprotein Cholesterol
MHE	Mental Health Enquiry
MOEH	Medical Officer of Environmental Health
MOH	Medical Officer of Health
MRC	Medical Research Council
OPCS	Office of Population Censuses and Surveys
OPV	Oral Polio Vaccine
OR	Odds Ratio
PHLS	Public Health Laboratory Service
PMR	Perinatal Mortality Rates
RCT	Randomized Controlled Trials
RHA	Regional Health Authority
SMR	Standardized Mortality Ratio
STD	Sexually Transmitted Disease
TLV	Threshold Limit Values

Part 1
Epidemiology

Chapter 1
General Principles

The word epidemiology is derived from Greek and means literally, studies upon people. Modern methods of epidemiological enquiry were first developed in the course of investigating outbreaks of infectious diseases in the nineteenth century. However, in contemporary medical practice the scope and applications of epidemiology have been greatly extended. Similar methods are now used in the investigation of the causes and natural history of all types of disease, as well as in the development and assessment of preventive programmes and treatments, and in the planning and evaluation of health services. In contrast to clinical medicine it involves the study of groups of people (populations) rather than the direct study of individuals. This in no way diminishes its relevance to clinical medicine. On the contrary, it enhances the practice of medicine by increasing the understanding of how diseases arise and how they might be managed both in the individual and in societies as a whole.

Most doctors from time to time find themselves involved with the subject in one way or another, either as participants in investigations or through the use they make of the results of epidemiological studies. It is, therefore, important that all doctors, and others involved in health care, should have an understanding of the subject so that they can take advantage of opportunities to use epidemiological methods in the study of health and disease and be able to evaluate other people's contributions before accepting their conclusions.

The investigation of causes and natural history of disease

One of the most important roles of epidemiology is to give a broader understanding of the causes and natural history of diseases than can ever be gained from the study of individuals. Clearly the experience of an individual clinician is limited because the number of patients with any particular problem with whom he or she comes into contact is relatively small. The less frequent a disease, the more fragmentary is an individual doctor's experience and understanding of it. If the experience of many doctors is recorded in a standard form and properly analysed then new and more reliable knowledge can often be acquired which will assist in diagnosis and point to optimum management policies. Such systematic collection and analysis of data about medical conditions in populations is the essence of epidemiology.

The value of pooling doctors' experience in elucidating the causes of disease is well illustrated by the story of the epidemic of fetal limb malformations (phocomelia) that was caused by taking the drug thalidomide during the first trimester of pregnancy. Phocomelia, a major deformity in the development of the limbs, was a recognized congenital abnormality long before the invention of thalidomide. A drawing by Goya called 'Mother with deformed child' bears witness to the fact that it occurred in eighteenth century Spain (Fig. 1.1). However, under normal circumstances it is a very rare abnormality. Doctors may encounter such rare conditions at some time during their professional life, but, because they know it has already been described, they are unlikely to regard a single case as a noteworthy observation. If, over a short period of time, each of a dozen or so doctors or midwives throughout the country delivered a child with such an abnormality, each would be personally interested. The significance of these individual cases would pass unnoticed unless they communicated with each other or there was a central reporting system. This is what happened early in the course of the thalidomide episode. One of the lessons learned from the episode was highlighted in the Chief Medical Officer's report of 1966. He said that it

> . . . focused attention on the lack of information concerning the different types of congenital malformations . . . Had a national scheme for notification been available at this time, it is probable that the increase in limb deformities would have been noticed earlier and perhaps some of the tragedies could have been avoided.

The thalidomide incident underlines the need to collect, collate and analyse data about the occurrence of disease in populations as a matter of routine. This will increase the probability that causes will be identified early and, whenever possible, eliminated. However, even with the most efficient and complete system of recording medical observations it is unlikely that all the problems of cause would be solved. It is interesting to speculate about what would have happened if thalidomide had been universally lethal to the fetus before the twelfth week of pregnancy. A large number of the 'spontaneous' abortions would have passed unnoticed, some even to the pregnant woman, and there might have been little or no indication that thalidomide had any deleterious effects on the human fetus. The discovery of such causal relationships requires other approaches, but still depends on the study of populations and cannot be established by examination of individual cases. The same is true for most proposed causes (agents) and other factors which may determine or predispose to the occurrence of disease.

Disease in perspective

Another application of epidemiological techniques is to give perspective to the range of diseases facing doctors and the diversity of their natural history. The individual clinician sees only a selected and comparatively small proportion of sick people, and so may gain an erroneous impression of the relative frequency of different conditions in the community as a whole. He may also fail to appreciate the range of different ways in which diseases present and progress. This is important since, consciously or not, the clinician tends to rely on his personal experience to assess the likelihood of particular diagnoses and the prognosis in his patients when deciding his management policy rather than on the broader experience of the profession as a whole. Only population surveys in which all cases of a condition in a defined population are identified and studied will allow an unbiased and comprehensive picture to emerge.

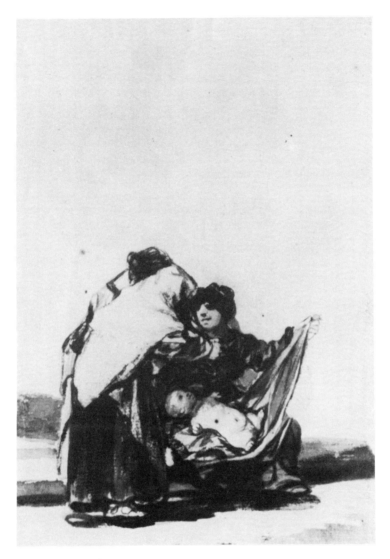

Fig. 1.1 'Mother with deformed child' by Francisco José Goya y Lucientes (by courtesy of the Cliché des Musées Nationaux, Paris).

Health care needs

Apart from its significance in day to day clinical practice, an unbalanced picture of disease incidence or prevalence may also distort a doctor's view of the health care needs of the community. Now, in the National Health Service and in most health care systems throughout the world, attempts are made to organize services according to priorities set by objective criteria rather than allowing them to be dictated solely by subjective judgments and traditional provision. An important report published in the early 1980s called 'Inequalities in Health' drew attention to some of the major differences that persist in the patterns of illness and disability in England and in the use of health services between different socioeconomic groups. For example, men in social class V were reported to suffer from 'long-standing' illnesses almost twice as often as those in social class I, but they consulted their family doctor only about 25% more often. This observation suggests a serious failure to match needs with appropriate services. It calls for detailed investigation of the relevant population groups to elucidate the reasons for it and the implications for future health care provision.

Evaluation of medical interventions

Finally, epidemiology is of value in testing the usefulness (and safety) of medical interventions. Although many existing remedies have never been subjected to trial, everyone nowadays recognizes the necessity to conduct clinical trials of a new drug or vaccine before it is introduced into medical practice. This is the only way to demonstrate that a particular drug or vaccine is likely to improve the patient's prospects of recovery or to prevent disease from occurring or progressing. Once a product has been launched on the market it is necessary to continue to monitor its effects (both beneficial and adverse) in order to ensure that patients are being prescribed effective and safe medication. In recent years pharmacoepidemiology, which is exclusively concerned with the application of epidemiological methods to the assessment of medicines, has been established.

It is now accepted that the same principles ought to be applied to other treatments such as surgery or physical therapy and even to the alternative ways in which health services can be provided. Such trials are becoming increasingly numerous, but they usually need to be on a large scale to produce reliable results. This is expensive and time consuming but necessary in the long-term interests of health services.

Clinical medicine and epidemiology

It will be clear from the above that there are important contrasts between the approaches to disease by clinicians and by epidemiologists. Recognition of these differences helps understanding of the subject.

The clinician asks the question 'What disease has my patient got?' The epidemiologist asks 'Why has this person rather than another developed the disease, why does the disease occur in winter rather than summer, or why in this country but not in another?' In order to answer these questions it is necessary to compare groups of people, looking for the factors that distinguish people with disease from those without the disease. Underlying the investigation of disease in this way is the belief that the misfortune of an individual in contracting it is not due to chance or fate but to a specific, definable and preventable combination of circumstances.

For a clinician, the utility of a diagnosis is as a pointer to management decisions. Therefore the diagnostic precision required is related to the specificity of treatments that are available. For an epidemiologist, diagnosis has different significance. It is a way of classifying individuals in order to make comparisons between groups. Lack of precision leads to poorly defined categories. This makes it difficult to identify the subtle yet important differences between groups which are critical to the understanding of the causes and prevention of disease.

The clinician is interested in the natural history of disease for prognostic purposes for an individual patient. He is usually content to express prognosis in terms such as 'good', 'bad', 'about 6 months', etc. It is unhelpful to him and his patient to attempt to introduce mathematical precision into prognostic statements such as, 'he has a 10.9% chance of surviving symptom-free for 5 years' though it may sometimes be appropriate to give a range of expected survival, for example between 3 and 7 years. By contrast, in population studies precision is helpful because it may allow the investigator to identify variables that have important effects on outcome. For example, it may be informative to investigate why in one group of patients 10.9% survive symptom-free for 5 years while in another group with approximately similar conditions, 26.5% survive symptom-free for 5 years. What accounts for this difference which could assist in planning treatment or preventive strategies?

While there are these clear differences between clinical and epidemiological approaches to medical problems and while their immediate purposes are different, it is also clear that the results of epidemiological investigations can contribute greatly to the scientific basis of clinical practice.

Chapter 2
Concepts of Cause and Risk and Types of Epidemiological Study

Introduction

The principal uses of epidemiology in medicine have been described in Chapter 1. These can be summarized as:

• *Firstly* the investigation of the causes and natural history of disease, with the aim of disease prevention and health promotion;

• *Secondly* the measurement of health care needs and the evaluation of clinical management, with the aim of improving the effectiveness and efficiency of health care provision.

Both involve two important and fundamental concepts—cause and risk. The concept of *cause* must be distinguished from the notion of association. Not all factors associated with the occurrence of disease are causes. They also include so-called 'determinants' and factors associated by chance. A *cause* is an external agent (microbe, chemical substance, physical trauma) which results in disease in susceptible individuals. A *determinant* is an attribute or circumstance that affects the liability of an individual to be exposed to or, when exposed, to develop disease, e.g. hereditary predisposition, environmental conditions.

The concept of *risk* includes both the 'risk' that a person exposed to a potentially harmful agent will develop a particular disease and the 'risk' that a particular intervention will beneficially or adversely influence the outcome. The indices commonly used to measure risk are set out below. *Risk factors* are different but are involved in both concepts. They are factors that are associated with a particular disease or outcome. They can be associated either by chance or because they influence the course of events. All causal agents and determinants are 'risk factors' but not all 'risk factors' are causal agents or determinants.

The purpose of epidemiological studies is to identify causes and to define and measure risks by the application of the scientific methods set out in the next four chapters.

CAUSES AND DETERMINANTS

Few diseases have a single 'cause'. Most are the result of exposure of susceptible individuals to one or more causal agents. Even in the case of some of the most straightforward illnesses, for example infections, exposure to the causal agent does not inevitably result in disease. Many other factors may influence the development of disease in addition to the direct cause. Thus the investigation of cause is usually a complex exercise that involves both the identification of the characteristics of susceptible individuals (and sometimes characteristics of individuals who appear to be unusually resistant) and the types of exposure to external agents that are necessary for the disease to occur.

Factors which are associated with the occurrence of a disease but which are not one of its causes are usually referred to as *confounding variables*. There are two broad types of confounding variable:

1   Factors which affect the individual's susceptibility or exposure to the causal agents (determinants). Many studies may show that a disease has a clear and statistically significant correlation with one or more of these factors. It is often of interest and value to identify them *but* the disease will not occur unless individuals are exposed to the underlying causal agent.

2   Factors that are independently associated both with the cause of the disease and with the disease itself but which are themselves the cause of neither. For example, heavy cigarette smoking and a high alcohol consumption tend to occur together. Smoking is causally associated with carcinoma of the bronchus and because heavy drinking is associated with cigarette smoking, alcohol consumption will tend to correlate with carcinoma of the bronchus.

Ideally causal hypotheses should be explored by carefully controlled experiments in which the effects of each of the postulated causes can be examined independently of other factors. In animal studies, for example, it is usually possible to exclude the effects of inheritance by breeding a family of animals for study. The possible effects of the general environment and diet that are not of interest for a particular investigation can be eliminated by rearing the whole family under standard conditions. Then the effects of a suspected causal agent can be assessed by exposing some of the animals to it whilst protecting others from it. In such experiments the only major differences between the two groups is their exposure to the agent under study. Such a study design allows the observed effects, if any, to be attributed unequivocally to the agent under investigation. It is impractical and unethical to undertake studies of such experimental purity amongst human subjects. The identification of the causes of diseases and factors that alter the course of a disease in humans, necessitates adopting methods whereby hypotheses can be tested without prejudice to the individuals being studied.

The methods that are used in epidemiological studies represent practical compromises of the above 'ideal' design. It is essential therefore that the results of any investigation are interpreted in full knowledge of the limitations imposed by the compromises. In particular it is important to take account of the effects of confounding variables and when these cannot be controlled in the study design, to allow for them in the analysis.

Distinguishing causes and determinants from chance association

As stated above, the observation that a disease is associated with a suspected agent is not proof that the suspected agent caused the disease. For example, there is a higher prevalence of alcoholism amongst publicans and barmen than in most other occupational groups. This does not necessarily mean that being a barman causes alcoholism. There are several other possible explanations of this phenomenon, including the fact that people who tend to excessive alcohol consumption may seek jobs in bars.

The types of evidence that can be used to distinguish a causal association from a fortuitous association are listed below. Many of the criteria appear to be simple and straightforward but it can be seen that each of them can present practical difficulties.

Time sequence

If an agent causes a disease then exposure must always precede its onset.

A practical problem is that it is often difficult to date exposure to a suspected causal agent and the date of onset of the disease. For example, AIDS is usually not manifest until many years after infection with HIV. Most people with AIDS could have become infected with HIV on many occasions. By the time the disease is apparent it is impossible to prove that a particular exposure or type of activity led to the infection.

Distribution of the disease

The spatial distribution of the disease should be similar to that of the suspected causal agent.

This may be difficult to demonstrate, particularly if there is a significant time interval between exposure and manifestation of disease *and* there have been movements in the population during that interval. For example, legionnaires disease commonly occurs in people who become infected as a result of casual or transient exposure to the source and who may be widely scattered before they develop symptoms of the disease.

Gradient

The incidence of disease should correlate with the amount and duration of exposure to the suspected cause (population dose–response).

For example, mesothelioma was noted to be more common than expected in asbestos workers and in those living near to factories which emitted asbestos dust into the atmosphere. The incidence was greatest in workers exposed for the longest periods and those living in closest proximity to the factories. In many instances it may be difficult to quantify exposure.

Consistency

The same association with a suspected causal agent should be found in studies in different populations.

Failure to find consistency may be explained by differences in study design. Caution is needed before rejecting a causal hypothesis in such circumstances. For example, studies designed to test the hypothesis that carcinoma of the breast is causally associated with exposure to oral contraceptives, have produced conflicting results. Some appear to demonstrate that women exposed to oral contraceptives over long periods of time have an increased risk of breast cancer under the age of 35 years; others do not support this hypothesis. Careful review of the studies reveals differences in the criteria for the selection of cases and in the analytic techniques used. A causal hypothesis can be regarded as supported only when there is a general consistency of findings from studies conducted in the same way.

Biological plausibility

The association between the disease and exposure to the suspected causal agent should be consistent with the known biological activity of the suspected agent.

Sometimes an association is observed before the biological process is identified. The fact that there is no *known* biological explanation for an association should not lead to the rejection of a biological hypothesis. For example, in the mid nineteenth century John Snow suggested that cholera was caused by an invisible agent in water. The epidemiological data were entirely consistent with the hypothesis but the cholera vibrio and its mode of spread had yet to be discovered.

Experimental models

The disease should be reproducible in experimental models with animals.

The fact that exposure to an agent can produce a disease in animals similar to that seen in man gives credence to a causal hypothesis, but failure to produce the disease amongst animals cannot be used as evidence to reject the hypothesis. For example, some micro-organisms are pathogenic in man but not usually in animals, e.g. measles virus; others are pathogenic in animals but not in man, and only a minority are normally pathogenic in both.

Preventive trials

Control or removal of the suspected agent results in decreased incidence of disease.

For example, when it was appreciated that the use of thalidomide for treatment of morning sickness in pregnancy was associated with a high incidence of phocomelia, the drug was withdrawn and the epidemic rapidly ceased.

RISK

There are three common indices of risk:
absolute;
relative;
attributable.

Absolute risk

This is the most basic measurement; it is the incidence rate of the disease amongst people exposed to an agent. This is not a very useful index because it assumes that no risk is incurred by people who are not exposed to the agent. For example, it is misleading to assess the dangers of oral contraceptives merely in terms of the mortality from diseases that might be associated with their use for two reasons. Firstly, the diseases that are associated with oral contraceptives are not exclusively caused by them (thrombo-embolic disease occurred in women before oral contraceptives were invented). Secondly, sexually active women who do not use oral contraceptives may either be exposed to a greater risk of pregnancy (and its consequent complications) or they may be exposed to the risks associated with another method of contraception, e.g. the IUD. It is therefore more useful to quantify the *relationship* between the risk of the disease amongst those exposed to the agent under investigation and those not so exposed.

Relative risk

This is the ratio of the incidence rate in the exposed group to the incidence rate in the non-exposed group. It is sometimes expressed as a percentage. It is a measure of the proportionate increase (or, if the agent is protective, the decrease) in disease rates of the exposed group. Thus it makes allowance for the frequency of the disease amongst people who are not exposed to the supposed harmful agent.

Attributable risk

This is the difference between the incidence rates in the exposed and the non-exposed groups, i.e. it represents the risk attributable to the factor being investigated.

The use of these measures of risk is illustrated with data collected during the course of a cohort study which compared mortality amongst cigarette smokers with non-smokers during a 7-year period (Table 2.1).

Table 2.1 A comparison of mortality amongst cigarette smokers and non-smokers.

	Number in study	Died within 7 years	Death rate over 7 years (per 1000)
Cigarette smokers	25 769	133	5.16
Non-smokers	5 439	3	0.55

Absolute risk in cigarette smokers = 5.16 per 1000
Relative risk in cigarette smokers = 5.16/0.55 = 9.38
Attributable risk in cigarette smoking = 5.16 − 0.55 = 4.61 per 1000

This indicates that smokers were 9.38 times more likely to die during the 7-year period than non-smokers and that the additional risk of death carried by smokers compared with non-smokers was 4.61 per thousand persons per 7-years. The confidence with which these findings can be applied to the general population is determined in part by the similarity of the groups in respect of attributes other than their smoking habits, in part upon whether the smokers are representative of the whole population of smokers and in part upon the sizes of the samples investigated. If the sampling was truly representative then the proportion of deaths attributable to smoking that would be eliminated by cessation of smoking, is the ratio of attributable to absolute risk (4.61/5.16 = 89%).

TYPES OF EPIDEMIOLOGICAL STUDY

There are three broad types of epidemiological study:

descriptive;

analytic;

intervention.

They serve different purposes. None of them is entirely clear cut and it is not profitable to try to classify each and every study within these three classical types. Frequently the detailed investigation of disease involves undertaking several studies of different types. They are defined and explained here to enable the reader to understand the concepts involved and to provide a framework which can be used to identify the most appropriate study to answer particular problems.

Descriptive studies

These are used to demonstrate the patterns in which diseases are distributed in populations. They aim to identify changes in mortality (deaths) and morbidity (illness) in time or to compare the incidence or prevalence of disease in different geographical areas or between groups of individuals with different characteristics (for example occupational groups). Correlations may then be sought with one or more other factors which may be thought to influence the occurrence of the diseases. Studies of this type may give rise to hypotheses of cause but cannot be used to explore the meaning of associations and can rarely prove cause. This requires the use of the other types of study.

Analytic studies

These are planned investigations designed to test specific hypotheses. They aim to define the causes or determinants of diseases more precisely than is possible using descriptive studies alone. From the results it is often possible to suggest ways whereby the disease may be prevented or controlled. There are two principal types of analytic study: *case-control* and *cohort*. They both rely on data collected in a systematic manner according to well defined procedures.

• In a *cohort* investigation individuals are selected for study either on the basis that they have been exposed to the agent under investigation or because they have some characteristic that makes them easy to investigate. They are 'followed-up' for a period of time that may extend into years in order to discriminate between those who develop the disease and those who do not.

• The subjects investigated in a *case-control* study are generally recruited because they already have the disease being investigated. Their past histories of exposure to suspected causal agents are compared with those of 'control' subjects, individuals who are not affected with the disease but are drawn from the same general population. The analysis involves discriminating between the past exposures of the cases and those of the controls.

The differences between these two study designs are schematically represented in Fig. 2.1. The cohort study design is closest to the 'ideal' experimental design. Such studies tend to take longer and to be more expensive than case-control studies. However they tend to yield more robust findings. Case-control studies are usually cheaper and quicker to complete but the results rarely give clear cut proof of cause.

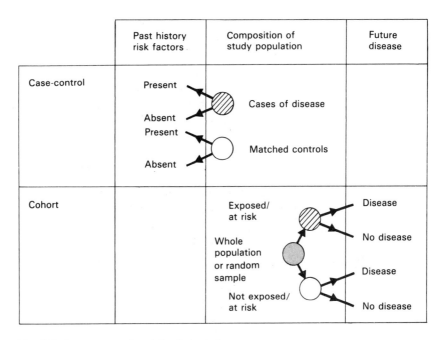

Fig. 2.1 Comparison of analytic study designs.

Intervention studies

These are essentially experiments designed to measure the efficacy and safety of particular types of health care intervention (treatment, prevention, control and the way in which health care is provided). They can also be used to assess the comparative effectiveness and efficiency of different interventions. The most familiar study design of this type is the clinical trial.

Definitions

Efficacy
This is a measure of the capacity of an intervention to produce a desired effect.

Effectiveness
This is a measure of the degree to which an intervention achieves its objective in practical use.

Efficiency
This is a measure of the comparative costs of different interventions in achieving the desired objective in practical use.

Chapter 3
Descriptive Studies

Introduction

An important starting point for many epidemiological investigations is the description of the patterns of distribution of disease in populations (descriptive studies). The principal advantages of descriptive studies are that they are cheap, quick to complete and they give a useful initial overview of a problem that may point to the next step in its investigation.

Usually descriptive studies make use of routinely collected health data, for example death certification data, hospital inpatient statistics or infectious disease notifications. The main sources of routine health data are set out in Chapter 8. The social and other variables in relation to which disease data may be examined are also available from a wide variety of routine sources. The actual source used for a particular investigation depends on the data that are required. With the exception of census material, routine sources of social data are not discussed in detail in this book.

Often the data required to describe disease distribution in a population and related variables are not readily available or are unsatisfactory for epidemiological purposes. In these circumstances it is necessary to conduct special surveys in order to collect the raw material for a descriptive study. These surveys are usually *cross-sectional* in type (see Chapter 4).

Uses of descriptive studies

Aetiological

The results of descriptive studies usually only give general guidance as to possible causes or determinants of disease, e.g. where broad geographical differences in prevalence are shown, but they may be quite precise, e.g. where a particular disease is very much more frequent within an occupational group. Analysis of the results may indicate that certain attributes or exposures are more commonly found amongst people who have the disease than in those who do not. The converse may also be demonstrated, namely that certain attributes are more commonly found amongst people who do not have the disease than in those who do. This may be an equally valuable finding. It is not possible to prove that an agent causes a disease from a descriptive study but investigations of this type will often generate or support hypotheses of aetiology and justify further investigations.

Clinical

Clinical impressions of the frequency of different conditions and their natural history are often misleading. The clinical impression is influenced by the special interests of individual doctors, by events that make a particular impression and by the chance clustering of cases. To obtain a balanced view of the relative importance of different conditions, their natural history and the factors that affect outcome requires data assembled from unbiased (random) samples of a total population. Precise knowledge of the relative frequency of different diseases at different times and in various situations and the normal distribution of physiological measurements in particular groups of persons is helpful to the clinician in his judgment of probabilities when deciding on the most likely diagnosis in individual patients.

Service planning

Health service planning in the past has been largely based on historical levels of provision and responses to demands for medical care. In order to plan services to meet needs rather than demand, and to allocate resources appropriately, accurate descriptive data are required on the relative importance and magnitude of different health problems in various segments of the community. It is also essential in order to evaluate the effectiveness of services provided and to monitor changes in disease incidence which may indicate a need for control action or the reallocation of resources and adjustments to service provision.

Analysis of descriptive data

Data derived from routine mortality and morbidity statistics (and from cross-sectional surveys) are usually analysed within three main categories of variable:
　　time (when?);
　　place (where?);
　　personal characteristics (who?).

Time

Three broad patterns of variation of disease incidence with time are recognizable. These are:
1　long-term (secular) trends;
2　periodic changes (including seasonality);
3　epidemics.

Long-term (secular) trends

These are changes in the incidence of disease over a number of years that do not conform to an identifiable cyclical pattern. For example, the secular trend in mortality from tuberculosis in England and Wales has shown a steady fall over many years (Fig. 3.1). The observation of this trend on its own does not give any indication of its cause. However, it is sufficiently striking to justify specific studies aimed at trying to identify the reasons for the change. The inclusion in the figure of the times at which various discoveries were made or specific measures were introduced gives some enlightenment. The overall trend seems to have been hardly affected by the identification of the causal organism, or the invention of streptomycin or by the introduction of BCG vaccination. This suggests that these played little part in the decline in mortality. However, the presentation of these

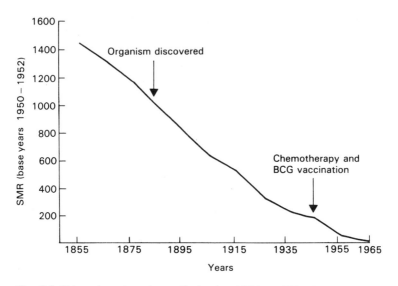

Fig. 3.1 Tuberculosis mortality in England and Wales 1855–1965 (arithmetic scale).

data on a simple arithmetic scale (as in Fig. 3.1) disguises an important feature of the trend, that is a change in the rate at which the decline occurred. When the data are plotted on a logarithmic scale (Fig. 3.2) it becomes clear that the introduction of specific measures for the control and treatment of tuberculosis was associated with an acceleration in the established decline in mortality. It is now thought that the decline in mortality from tuberculosis was due to a complex series of changes. Until the 1950s these were mainly an increase in the resistance of the population to infection and environmental changes that reduced the chances of acquiring infection. After the early 1950s the decline in the mortality rate was accelerated by the newly available methods of management.

It is frequently necessary to examine secular trends both as changes in rates (arithmetic scale) and as rates of change (logarithmic scale) if the nature of a trend is to be fully appreciated.

The secular trend in mortality from carcinoma of the bronchus shows the opposite picture to that for tuberculosis (Fig. 3.3). Until quite recently it had been increasing relentlessly amongst males but the rate of increase has now declined. By contrast the increase in mortality rates amongst women continues. The trend in male mortality shows a powerful correlation with changes in the national consumption of cigarettes. This observation gave rise to the hypothesis that cigarette smoking could be the causal agent, although it does not prove causality. The hypothesis has since been explored through large numbers of analytic and intervention studies.

Periodic changes

These are more or less regular or cyclic changes in incidence, the most common examples of which are seen in infectious diseases. For example, until a vaccine was introduced, measles showed a regular biennial cycle in incidence in England

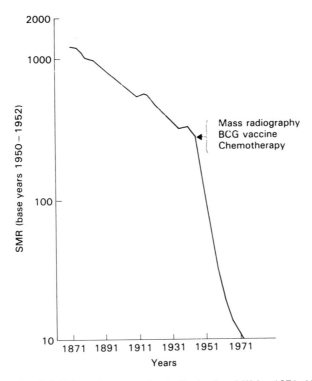

Fig. 3.2 Tuberculosis mortality in England and Wales 1871–1971 (logarithmic scale). (Reproduced with permission from HMSO: Prevention & Health: Everybody's Business 1976.)

and Wales (Fig. 3.4). The cycles were probably the result of changes in the levels of child population (herd) immunity (see pp. 116–117). Other infectious diseases such as whooping cough, rubella and infectious hepatitis show less regular, but nevertheless distinct, cycles with longer intervals between peaks.

Seasonality

This is a special example of periodic change. The environmental conditions that favour the presence of an agent and the likelihood of its successful transmission change with the seasons of the year. Respiratory infections, which spread directly from person to person by the airborne route, are more common in winter months when people live in much closer contact with each other than in the summer. By contrast, gastrointestinal infections, which spread by the faecal–oral route, often through contamination of food, are more common in summer months when the ambient temperatures favour the multiplication of bacteria in food. The regular seasonality of gastrointestinal infections is shown in Fig. 3.5 which plots the number of notifications of food poisoning for each quarter in 1974–1989. A particularly interesting feature of food poisoning incidence is that the marked seasonality is combined with a noticeable secular trend. The numbers of cases notified in late 1988 and early 1989 was much

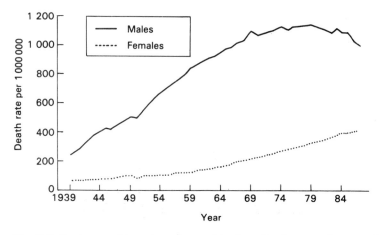

Fig. 3.3 Carcinoma of lung, bronchus and trachea. Deaths per million population in England and Wales. NB: changes in classification in 1950 and 1963.

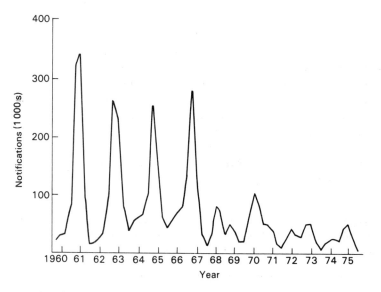

Fig. 3.4 Quarterly notifications of measles in England and Wales 1960–1975.

higher than in previous years. This could be due to the contamination in the food chain, a decline in standards of food storage, distribution or preparation, or the result of an increase in notification rates following publicity given to the problem of food poisoning.

Some non-infectious conditions, e.g. allergic rhinitis, deaths from drowning and road accidents, also display distinct seasonality. For most of these the explanation for the seasonality is not difficult to infer. There are seasonal variations in the incidence of certain other conditions, however, for which there is as yet no rational explanation. For example, schizophrenics are more likely

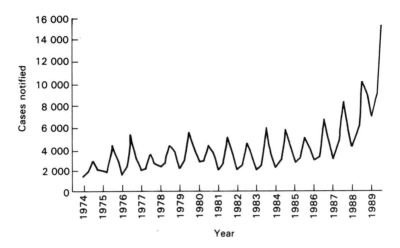

Fig. 3.5 Quarterly notifications of food poisoning in England and Wales, 1974–1989.

than the general population to be born in the early months of the year (February and March) (Table 3.1). Many hypotheses have been offered to explain this observation, including the proposition that the disease is caused by an intrauterine infection, that the mothers of schizophrenics are more likely to miscarry at certain times of the year (thereby resulting in a deficit of births in months other than February and March) and that the mothers of schizophrenics are more likely to conceive in April and May than are other women. However, none has yet been proved.

It should be noted that the seasonality in disease patterns related to climatic conditions is reversed in the southern hemisphere.

Table 3.1 Seasonality of birth of schizophrenics and neurotics compared with that of the general population (expected) showing an increased frequency of births of schizophrenics in the first part of the year but no seasonality amongst neurotics. (Adapted from Hare E, Price J, Slater E. *Br J Psychiat* 1974; **124**: 81–86.)

	Quarter of birth			
	Jan–Mar	Apr–June	July–Sept	Oct–Dec
Schizophrenics				
Observed	1383	1412	1178	1166
Expected	1292.1	1342.8	1293.1	1211.1
Observed as a percentage of expected	107	105	91	96
Neurotics				
Observed	3085	3172	2949	2882
Expected	3024.1	3150.6	3042.0	2844.2
Observed as a percentage of expected	101	101	97	101

Epidemics

These are temporary increases in the incidence of disease in populations. The most obvious epidemics are of infectious diseases such as influenza (Fig. 3.6) but non-infectious epidemics do occur. For example, there was an increase in asthma deaths in the 1960s associated with the increased use of pressurized aerosol bronchodilators (Fig. 3.7).

The word 'epidemic' is also sometimes used to describe an increase in incidence above the level expected from past experience in the same population (or from experience in another population with similar demographic and social characteristics). However, if the strict definition of epidemics is used, it is inappropriate to use the term to describe recent secular trends in coronary heart disease, lung cancer or even AIDS since there is no evidence that any of them are temporary increases in incidence.

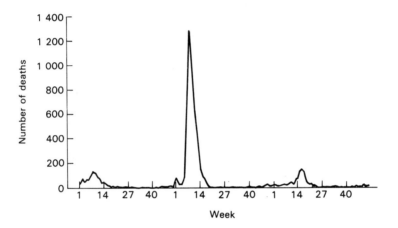

Fig. 3.6 Weekly deaths from influenza in England and Wales 1975–1977.

Place

Variations in the incidence or prevalence of disease by place can be considered under three headings:

broad geographical differences;
local differences;
variations within single institutions (e.g. factory, residential home or hospital).

Broad geographical differences

Variations in the incidence of disease are sometimes related to factors such as climate, social and cultural habits (including diet), the presence of vectors or of other naturally occurring hazards. Although the incidence of disease does not respect administrative boundaries between countries or regions, these boundaries often follow broadly natural ecological boundaries and tend to encompass common social and cultural groups. Much valuable information pointing to possible causes of disease has been obtained by the careful analysis of data

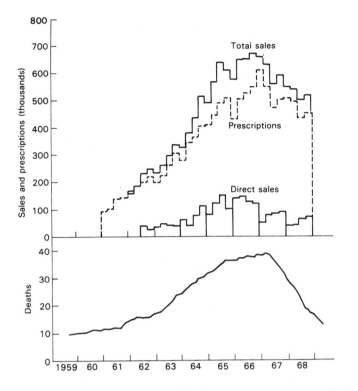

Fig. 3.7 Sales and prescriptions of asthma preparations compared with deaths from asthma among people aged 5–34 years, in England and Wales 1959–1968. (After Inman W H W, Adelstein A M. *Lancet* 1969; **ii**: 279.)

collected routinely within countries and other administrative units. For example, various forms of cancer and other conditions show striking geographical difference in incidence (Table 3.2).

Local differences

The distribution of a disease may be limited by the localization of its cause. Thus, if a main water supply becomes contaminated, the illnesses that result from the contamination will be clustered in people living within the distribution area of the water. 'Spot-maps' on which cases are marked, may show local concentrations which suggest possible sources. In interpreting such maps it is important to relate the spatial distribution of cases to the density of population. The classical study of the 1854 cholera outbreak in the Golden Square area of London by John Snow used such a technique and led him to identify the particular water pump that was the source of the infection. In this instance, cases were clustered in the streets close to the Board Street pump, while comparatively few cases occurred in the vicinity of other pumps in the area.

A special kind of locality difference is that which exists between *urban* and *rural* environments. In general, people who live in urban areas are subjected to

Table 3.2 Geographical variation in the incidence of disease. Comparison of death rates in England and Wales with those in Japan (1979) for various causes shows considerable discrepancies. Both are highly industrialized countries with well developed health services, but have very different cultures and racial origins (data from *World Health Statistics Annual*, WHO, Geneva 1981).

	Disease	(Rates per 100 000)	
		England and Wales	Japan
England and Wales high Japan low	Cancer of breast (females)	47.9	6.6
	Cancer of prostate	20.2	2.9
	Cancer of colon	20.9	6.3
England and Wales low Japan high	Cancer of stomach	23.0	43.8
	Cirrhosis of liver (males)	5.0	21.1
	Suicide	8.5	18.0

different hazards from those experienced by people who live in rural areas. These differences alter their risk of certain diseases, sometimes to the advantage of the country person and sometimes to the benefit of the town dweller. In urban areas there may be better housing and sanitation but more overcrowding and air pollution; more leisure but less exercise, fresh food and sunlight; more industrial hazards but fewer risks of infection from animal contacts and vectors. In industrial societies, however, where commuting is a common practice, the distinction between town and country dwellers is often blurred. Table 3.3 shows some differences in mortality between urban and rural areas in England and Wales.

Variations within single institutions

In institutions such as schools, military barracks, holiday camps and hospitals, variations in attack rates by class, platoon, chalet or ward may focus attention on

Table 3.3 Differences in mortality amongst males between urban and rural districts in England and Wales 1969–73 (SMRs).

		Urban with populations:			
	Conurbations	Over 100 000	50 000– 100 000	Under 50 000	Rural
Malignant neoplasms of bronchus, trachea and lung	118	109	98	90	79
Bladder	112	109	99	96	82
Chronic rheumatic heart disease	114	110	88	94	85
Ischaemic heart disease	99	106	107	101	95
Influenza	84	98	90	116	111
Bronchitis	117	109	98	96	76
Motor vehicle accidents	87	95	98	99	124
Accidental poisoning	126	110	100	89	67
Homicide	151	99	95	71	56

possible sources or routes of spread. For example, in an outbreak of surgical wound infection, identifying the bed positions of patients, ward duties of staff and theatres used may suggest the identity of a carrier or other source of infection. Similarly, in places of work the danger of developing disease may be shown to be inversely related to distance from source of a chemical hazard.

A high incidence of a disease amongst people who share the same environment does not prove that a factor within the environment was the cause of the disease. It may be that the people have chosen, or have been chosen, to share the same environment because they have an increased susceptibility to that disease or because of pre-existing disease or disability.

Persons

The chances of an individual developing a disease are affected by personal characteristics. The analysis of data on the incidence of disease in relation to the personal characteristics of victims, provides useful indicators of possible causes. The personal characteristics can be classified as:

intrinsic factors which affect susceptibility if exposed;

personal habits (or lifestyle) which affect exposure to causal agents.

Intrinsic factors

Age

Most diseases vary in both frequency and severity with age. In general, children are more susceptible to infectious diseases, young adults are more accident prone and older adults tend to suffer the results of long exposure to occupational and other environmental hazards. In infancy, immaturity and genetic defects affect susceptibility to disease. In later life, physiological changes, degenerative processes and an increased liability to malignant tumours are the dominant determinants of the patterns of illness.

The fact that the incidence of most diseases varies with age can complicate the comparison of morbidity and mortality between populations with dissimilar age structures. For example, the age structure of a population of military personnel is likely to be substantially different from that of a group of practising physicians. Therefore, it is to be expected that the two groups will differ in their incidence of many diseases. In order to make a valid comparison between these populations it is essential to adjust the data to take account of differences in their age structure. This procedure is called standardization, see p. 76.

Age differences in the incidence of disease may also be accounted for by a so-called *cohort effect*. This occurs when individuals born in a particular year, or living at a particular point in time, were exposed to the same noxious agent. They then carry an enhanced risk of the disease caused by that noxious agent for a long period, sometimes for the rest of their lives. For example, the children who were exposed to radiation in Hiroshima and Nagasaki in 1945 when the atomic bombs were detonated have had higher than expected incidence of leukaemia throughout their lives.

Sex

There is evidence that males are intrinsically more vulnerable to disease and death than are females. This is first apparent in the differential rates of still birth and early neonatal mortality and remains throughout life (Table 3.4). Indeed, during later life, with the exception of disorders that are specific to the female, there are few diseases which have a greater incidence in women than in men. In most societies men are exposed to a greater number and variety of hazards than are females often because of differences in their leisure and work activities. Even when the two sexes are exposed to the same hazards for the same period of time, there is evidence that women are less likely to develop disease and that they survive better than men. Some diseases appear to vary in incidence between the sexes only because they are more readily diagnosed in one sex than the other, e.g. gonorrhoea, or because they are more likely to come to medical attention, e.g. in mothers of young children.

Marital status

Morbidity and mortality from many diseases vary considerably according to marital status. In most cases both are higher amongst single persons. There are two reasons for this. Firstly, marriage is not random. People with pre-existing handicaps or disease are less likely to marry than those without. Thus individuals so affected will be over represented in the single (never married) population. Secondly, there are differences between the lifestyles of married and non-married people which affect their exposure to causal agents, for example sexual behaviour, contact with children, leisure activity and diet.

The incidence of some diseases and health problems is higher amongst divorced and widowed people than amongst married people, e.g. suicide and certain types of mental illness. It is always important to distinguish diseases and exposures that may have determined the marital status of an individual from those that are determined by the marital status.

Table 3.4 Death rates at different ages for males and females in England and Wales, 1988. (Deaths per 1000.)

Age	Males	Females
Still births	5.35	4.68
Under 28 days	5.81	4.39
Under 1 year	5.50	3.87
1–4 years	0.44	0.40
5–14 years	0.22	0.17
15–24 years	0.77	0.31
25–34 years	0.87	0.47
35–44 years	1.67	1.12
45–54 years	5.27	3.23
55–64 years	16.60	9.25
65–74 years	42.89	23.44
75–84 years	101.07	62.53
85 years +	214.71	171.00

Ethnic group

This term tends to be used very loosely to describe a number of personal characteristics, including some that are strictly genetically determined, e.g. skin colour, and some that have nothing to do with genetics, e.g. country of birth and religion. It is often difficult to disentangle these 'ethnic' characteristics from a number of other factors which affect the incidence of disease, e.g. dietary habits, religious practices, occupation and socioeconomic status. The effect of ethnicity on the incidence of disease is best studied in communities where people of different groups are living side by side and in similar circumstances. Some studies have been undertaken in Israel and in the USA in which very marked differences in the severity and frequency of disease between ethnic groups have been demonstrated. For example, in the USA cancer of the cervix has been shown to be much more common in black people than in white, whereas cancer of the breast is more common in white people than in black. It is always important to establish whether differences in disease incidence between people of different races are genetically or environmentally determined.

Personal habits or lifestyle

Family

Some diseases are especially frequent in certain families because of a common genetic inheritance, which is an intrinsic characteristic of the individuals. The risk of disease among members of the same family may also be increased because the members share a common environment and culture. Culture affects a wide range of disease-related factors such as type of housing, dietary habits and the way in which food is prepared, as well as the individual's reaction to illness.

Occupation and socioeconomic group

Some people are exposed to special risks in the course of their occupation. These include exposures to dust (particularly coal dust, silica and asbestos), toxic substances and gases used in industrial processes, and the risks of accident. Some occupations influence habits such as the amount of tobacco smoked and of alcohol consumed or the regularity of meals, which in turn affect disease incidence.

When interpreting any observed correlation between occupation and disease it is necessary to take account of the factors which determine a person's choice of occupation. Some may affect the person's susceptibility to disease, for example — tall and powerful people may choose physically demanding occupations whilst others may chose 'sheltered' occupations because they already suffer mentally or physically disabling diseases. Some, because of chronic disease, may be unable to keep demanding jobs in the higher socioeconomic groups; they tend to move down the social scale (social class migration).

The *social class* of men and single women is defined in terms of their occupation and their status within an occupational group (i.e. manager, foreman, unskilled). The social class of married women and of children is determined by the occupation of the husband (father). The concept of social class encompasses income group, education, and social status, as well as occupation. Most diseases show a positive social class gradient, with a higher incidence in manual workers than in professional groups (Table 3.5).

Interactions of time, place and personal characteristics

Frequently two or more factors correlate with the incidence of a disease and also with each other. It may be that only one factor is a causal agent or determinant and that the correlation with a second factor is fortuitous. Sometimes, however, two separate causes of disease interact with each other in such a way that the effect of the two acting together in the same individuals is greater than that of either acting alone. For example, while asbestos workers who do not smoke have a higher incidence of bronchial carcinoma than other non-smokers, those who smoke have a much higher incidence than would be expected in persons with similar smoking habits in the general population. Interactions such as this are often very complex and the analysis of observed distributions can do no more than indicate possible determinants which merit more detailed and carefully controlled enquiry.

Time, place and person interactions can be separated if circumstances arise in which one of the variables can be kept constant while the others change. For example, comparison of disease frequency in migrant populations with that in their place of origin is often informative, particularly where migrants move from an area with a high incidence of disease to one with a low incidence or vice versa. When they migrate they take with them their original hereditary susceptibilities but they change their risk of exposure to harmful agents. For example, the incidence of cancer of the stomach is higher in Japanese living in Japan than those living in the USA, while for cancer of the large bowel the reverse is true. In time, when migrants are assimilated into the host- culture, they may be

Table 3.5 Standardized mortality ratios for ages 15–64 years (England and Wales) showing trends by social class for specific causes of death.

| Cause of death (ICD number) | SMR by social class | | | | | |
	I	II	IIIN	IIIM	IV	V
Malignant neoplasm of stomach (151)	50	66	79	118	125	147
Malignant neoplasm of trachea, bronchus and lung (162)	53	68	84	118	123	143
Ischaemic heart disease (410–414)	88	91	114	107	108	111
Cerebrovascular disease (430–438)	80	86	98	106	111	136
Bronchitis, emphysema and asthma (490–493)	36	51	82	113	128	188

exposed to new risks in that culture. Thus studies of migrant groups can also be used to measure the latent period between exposure and onset of disease. For example, the incidence of multiple sclerosis is higher in Europeans who migrated to South Africa before the age of 15 than in those born in South Africa.

It must be stressed that caution is needed in studies of migrants because they are self-selected from the original population and their risks of disease may have been different from those who did not migrate.

Chapter 4
Surveys and Survey Methods

Introduction

Many descriptive studies make use of routinely collected data. However, such data are often unsatisfactory for this purpose and specifically designed surveys are needed. The problems with routine data include:

Difficulties in ascertainment of cases;
Variations in diagnostic criteria;
Absence of records of individual attributes;
Unsuitable format of records;
Inconsistency in data presentation.

Difficulties in ascertainment of cases

The recorded number of patients with a condition may vary for reasons that have nothing to do with the actual frequency of the disease. For example, the tendency to seek medical attention and the availability of services may vary. This source of bias is of greatest importance when studying illnesses that are rarely fatal, and therefore do not appear on death certificates or that are not always medically managed or reported and therefore do not come to the attention of the medical profession.

Example

Oesteoarthritis is neither fatal nor is it always treated or reported. Studies of that disease based entirely on the cases treated in hospital or brought to the attention of the general practitioner are misleading.

Variations in diagnostic criteria

These tend to vary between doctors and may change with time. This may be simply a matter of fashion or because the facilities for accurate diagnosis vary. Sometimes there may be agreed changes in classification practices from time to time and place to place.

Example

The International Classification of Diseases (ICD) is revised about every 10 years and some categories may not be carried forward from one edition to the next.

In addition the diagnosis may involve a measurement that is not made routinely and/or recorded for the whole (or a random sample) of the population.

Example

It is extremely difficult to study the epidemiology of hypertension in the community without doing special surveys because blood pressure is not a measurement that is routinely recorded in the population as a whole. By contrast, birth weight can be studied in some detail because all newly born babies are weighed and their weight is usually recorded.

Absense of records of individual attributes

The attributes of the individuals which it is proposed to investigate in relation to the presence of disease may not be recorded systematically.

Example

The occupation of patients is often not recorded or not recorded in sufficient detail in hospital notes to allow investigation of a cancer which it is suspected may result from occupational exposure to a carcinogenic agent.

Unsuitable format of records

The data are recorded but are not usable for studies because the form of the record is unsuitable, or because they are governed by strict rules of confidentiality.

Example

Diagnoses may be recorded but not in a form or in sufficient detail to allow classification by ICD or other standard criteria.

Inconsistency in data presentation

In the analysis of deaths the numbers and the date of occurrence are indisputable in countries where death registration is standard practice. However, when analysing morbidity by time, there are several possible points of reference. Those commonly used are the date of onset of the disease, the date of onset of symptoms, the date of first diagnosis or the date of hospital admission. In acute diseases, where these points are close together, it does not matter very much which is chosen, but in the case of chronic diseases the intervals may be months or even years. In such circumstances the reference point must be stated and be consistent.

The above difficulties with routinely available data can be partly overcome by well designed routine information systems. Nevertheless this cannot meet all requirements and many of the problems can only be overcome by surveys in which the data and means of collection are specified in advance and in which the study population is clearly defined.

Cross-sectional (prevalence) surveys

A cross-sectional (prevalence) survey is simply a descriptive study in which, instead of relying on routine sources of data, uses data collected in a planned way from a defined population. The aim is to describe individuals in the population at a particular point in time in terms of their personal attributes and their history of exposure to suspected causal agents. These data are then examined in relation to the presence or absence of the disease under investigation or its severity with a view to developing or testing hypotheses as described in Chapter 3.

Example
A survey of chronic bronchitis amongst London post office workers was carried out by Fletcher and colleagues in the 1950s. They studied 192 men and 192 women aged 40–59 years. The subjects were asked about their respiratory symptoms, history of respiratory illnesses and their smoking habits; their sputum volume and ventilatory capacity were measured and their sickness absence records were inspected. The study showed that chronic cough and phlegm production were significantly more common in men than in women and that symptoms in men, but not in women, increased in prevalence with age. The prevalence of symptoms and of a history of chest illness also increased steeply in relation to the amount of tobacco smoked. Impairment of ventilatory capacity was significantly correlated in men with the production of sputum, smoking and a history of chest illness (Fig. 4.1).

Comment
The demonstration of these associations in a population sample were important in confirming observations made amongst chronic bronchitics in clinical practice. However, this study on its own could not be used to unravel the sequence of events that lead to the development of disease. It could not show, for example, whether smoking predisposed individuals to chest illnesses which in turn

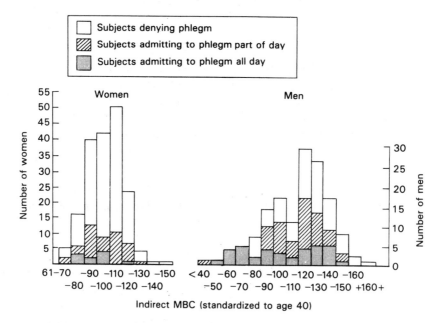

Fig. 4.1 Distribution of age standardized indirect maximum breathing capacity (MBC) (litres per minute). (From Fletcher C M, Elmes P C, Fairbain A S, Wood C H. *Br Med J* 1959; **2**: 257.)

damaged respiratory function, or whether chest illnesses increased the individuals' susceptibility to the harmful effects of smoking. These questions could only be answered with cohort studies (see p. 38).

Problems with survey methods

A number of practical and theoretical problems can arise in the design and conduct of cross-sectional surveys and other studies which may invalidate the results unless handled properly. The investigator needs to be aware of these potential problems and familiar with the methods that are available to solve them or to minimize their effects.

Sampling

It is usually unnecessary to study the whole of a population in order to obtain useful and valid information about that population. The investigation of a sample has many practical advantages. In particular it reduces the number of individuals who have to be interviewed, examined or investigated. It is also often easier to obtain high response rates and good quality information on smaller numbers. This is always preferable to poor quality data on larger numbers. If a sample is used it is essential to ensure that the individuals included in the sample are genuinely representative of the population being investigated, the 'parent' population. There are many methods available for selecting a sample and the method chosen depends upon the nature of the investigation that is being conducted. Some commonly used sampling techniques are:

Simple random sample

This is one in which each individual in the parent population has an equal chance (probability) of being selected. One way of obtaining a random sample is to give each individual a number and then to use a table of random numbers to decide which individuals should be included. Another method, which is more convenient and is adequate for most purposes, is to select people at regular intervals from a list of the total population. This is called a *systematic sample* and it has the advantage of being easy for field workers to use.

Example

If a one in ten sample of school children is required then every tenth child on the school role could be included. In some circumstances this method can lead to bias, e.g. when the school roll (or similar list) is compiled by class (or other grouping) which may affect randomness.

Stratified sample

This is one in which the probability of an individual being included varies according to a known and predetermined characteristic. The aim of this method is to ensure that small sub-groups which are of particular interest to the investigator are adequately represented.

Example

If one of the attributes being investigated in a cross-sectional study of school children is the consequences of being an immigrant to the country and immigrants comprise 5% of the population, then a simple random sample would produce a group in which 5% are immigrants. Unless the sample is very large, the number in the group may be insufficient for a conclusive analysis. To avoid this problem the sample has to be *weighted* in favour of the selection of immigrant children. This is done by drawing separate random samples from amongst immigrant and indigenous children, e.g. 50% of immigrants and 10% of the indigenous group. Thus all immigrant and all indigenous children have equal chances of selection although the chance of an immigrant being selected is greater than the chance of a locally born child being selected. When the data are analysed the fact that the sample was recruited in this way must be taken into account.

Cluster sample

This involves the use of groups as the sampling unit rather than individuals, e.g. households, school classes or residents within blocks on grid map. The groups to be studied should be randomly selected from all possible groups of the same type, e.g. a random sample of all households in England as in the General Household Survey undertaken routinely by OPCS. All members of the selected groups are included in the study. The underlying assumption is that the individuals belonging to any particular group do so for reasons unconnected with the disease being studied and the presence of any factor under investigation. The main advantage of this method of sampling is that the field work is concentrated and, therefore, simpler and cheaper. The principal disadvantage is that diseases and associated factors themselves may have determined the group to which individuals belong which the investigator may not suspect.

Multistage sampling

This combines all the above sampling techniques. For example, a series of 'clusters' say schools, are identified and a random sample of them is selected. Then within each school, a random sample of pupils stratified by class is recruited to the study.

Bias in sampling

There are four important potential sources of bias in selecting any sample:

1. Any deviation from the rules of selection can destroy the randomness of the sample. One of the most common temptations is to recruit volunteers to the study. This is in effect self-selection of participants and such individuals tend to be unrepresentative of the parent population.

2. Bias is introduced if people who are hard to identify in the parent population under study are omitted from the study. Thus, in investigating the health of school children the omission of children who are persistent absentees may seriously bias results if the reason for their absence is chronic illness.

3. The replacement of previously selected individuals by others can easily introduce bias. If, for example, it proves difficult to trace a person who has been selected or if that person refuses to cooperate, it is not acceptable to replace him or her with an easily traceable or cooperative individual. Replacement of a selected individual is acceptable only if it transpires that a selected individual was sampled in error, e.g. the list of eligible people was out of date or a selected subject was subsequently found not to satisfy study criteria.

4. If large numbers of individuals in the sample refuse to cooperate in a study the results may be meaningless. Therefore, it is essential to make intensive efforts to enlist the cooperation of and trace all the individuals who have been sampled.

Errors in rates

The analysis of epidemiological survey data usually entails the calculation of rates, e.g. incidence and prevalence rates, in exposed and non-exposed population groups. Rates may be affected by errors and bias in either the numerator or the denominator or both. Such errors can invalidate comparisons between rates and result in misleading conclusions.

Errors and bias in numerator data

The quality of numerator data is crucial for accurate classification of individuals according to their personal attributes and exposure to suspected causal agents and according to whether or not they have the disease under investigation. In contrast to descriptive studies based on routine data, special surveys offer the investigator the advantage of being able to specify the observations that he or she wishes to be made, rather than being constrained by the data that are collected for other purposes. Furthermore, the investigator can prescribe the methods to be used in examining or questioning the individuals involved in the study. However, the investigator usually only has a single opportunity to make the observations on each subject. It is therefore essential that the information required is clearly defined at the outset and that efforts are made to ensure that consistent results are obtained by the instruments (questionnaires, laboratory or other measuring equipment) used. Without clarity of definition in the design of the study and consistency in its execution, errors will occur.

Errors and bias in numerator data can be considered under the following headings:

subject variation;
observer variation;
limitations of the technical methods used.

Subject variation

Differences in observations made on the same subject on different occasions may be due to many factors, including those outlined below.

- Physiological changes in the parameter observed, e.g. blood pressure, blood glucose.
- Factors affecting the response to a question, e.g. recollection of past events, motivation to respond and mood at time of interview, reaction to environment and rapport with interviewer.

- Induced changes because the subject is aware that he or she is being studied.

Observer variation

The principal types of observer variation are:

- Failure of the same observer to record the same result on repeated examination of the same material (inconsistency). This is called *intra-observer* variation.
- Failure of different observers to record the same result. This is called *inter-observer* variation. The greater the number of different observers the greater are the chances of variation between them.

Either of the above types of error can arise for several reasons.

- Bias induced by awareness of the hypothesis under investigation, e.g. subjects' response to questions about exposure to 'risk factors' such as sexual orientation in a study of HIV infection, or observers' inclination to diagnose disease or to probe answers to questions in an investigation of adverse reactions to a drug or vaccine.
- Errors in executing the test or variations in the phrasing of a question, e.g. failure to be consistent in the use of a procedure, carelessness in setting up instruments or reading a scale, failure to follow instructions when administering a questionnaire, omission of some questions or tests, errors in recording of results.
- Lack of experience or skill and idiosyncrasies of observers, especially when classification depends on a subjective assessment, e.g. misinterpretation by the interviewer of an answer to a question, lack of skill in the manipulation of instruments, poor motivation and interest in the project.
- Bias in the execution of the test, e.g. preconception of what is 'normal' or 'to be expected', digit preference, i.e. tendency to 'round off' readings to whole numbers, fives and tens, inflection of voice in asking questions.

Limitations of the technical methods used

Technical methods may give incorrect or misleading results due to the following reasons.

- The test is inappropriate, i.e. it does not measure what it is intended to measure, e.g. the presence of albuminuria in pregnancy, for which there are many causes, is a poor index on its own of the presence of toxaemia. Therefore, a study of toxaemia in which cases are identified solely by albuminuria will give misleading results.
- The method used is intrinsically unreliable or inaccurate, i.e. the results are not repeatable, correspond poorly with those obtained by alternative methods, or do not correlate well with the severity of the condition being measured, e.g. peak flow rate in asthma.
- Faults in the test system, e.g. defective instruments, erroneous calibration, poor reagents, etc.

Avoidance of error and bias

There are no hard and fast rules that can be applied to ensure that errors do not arise in surveys and that bias is avoided. Each project will require careful thought and consideration of where errors and bias might arise. Some of the more straightforward principles are given below.

• The criteria used in *diagnostic classification* must be clearly defined and rigidly adhered to (even at the risk of missing a few cases). The features that must be present (or absent) for a diagnosis to be made must be specified.

• *Classification of severity or grade of disease* should be in quantitative terms where possible and it should cover the full range of possible types of case.

• All *subjects* should be observed under similar biological conditions on each occasion. Avoid uncomfortable circumstances. Design simple questions and use check questions for consistency of response.

• The number of *observers* used should be kept to a minimum. They should be trained properly to enhance their skills and test their variation on dummy subjects (or specimens). Take duplicate readings and record the mean value. Arrange reassessment of classification by different observers, e.g. X-ray films, stage of disease.

• Where possible, subjects and observers should be unaware of (blinded to) the specific hypothesis under investigation in order that they are not influenced by personal perceptions of the significance of the variables being recorded.

• The *tests* selected should be relevant to the purpose. Those that give the most consistent results and are least disturbing to the subject are preferable.

• *Equipment* should be simple, reliable and easy to use.

• *Test methods* should be standardized by, for example, the use of standard reagents, sets of graded X-rays or slides, standard wording of questions and instructions on probing and interpretation of answers, calibration of instruments against a standard reference. Quality control should be maintained to avert 'drift' from standards.

Denominator errors

Denominator errors occur when the population being investigated is not fully defined or when not all the eligible subjects are investigated. They can be minimized, firstly, by making every effort to encourage cooperation of the subjects by avoiding any inconvenience or discomfort to them. Secondly, all available means should be used to trace and persuade non-attenders to take part or continue to participate. The similarity of those who participate and those who are lost should be checked by comparing their general attributes such as age, marital status, sex and occupation to establish how representative they are of the total sample.

There are several ways of handling people *lost to follow-up* in the analysis phase of an investigation.

• Exclude them from both the numerator and the denominator.

• Include them up to the time that they left. This involves calculating units of 'time at risk' (see p. 39).

• Include all those 'lost' for half the 'time at risk' on the assumption that the rate of loss was even throughout the period and on average each individual was present for half the time.

• Analyse the data on the assumption that all those lost developed the disease, or had the most adverse outcome, and then on the assumption that none of them developed it. This will show the range within which the true result might lie.

Assessment of error in surveys

Some terms that are frequently used in the assessment of error in surveys are given below.

Random error

This is due to the chance fluctuation of recorded values around the 'true' value of an observation.

Systematic error (bias)

This is a consistent difference between the recorded value and the 'true' value in a series of observations. For example, if the height of an individual is always measured when the person is wearing shoes, then the measurement will be consistent but will have a systematic bias.

Discrimination

The aim of a test is either to separate persons with a disease (or a particular attribute) from those without the disease (or attribute) or to place subjects accurately on a range of severity (or a scale measuring an attribute). The degree to which this is achieved correctly is a measure of discrimination. A test with good discriminatory power has a small range of error in relation to the potential range of true results. There are two basic characteristics of a test which measure its discriminatory powers: its reproducibility and its validity.

Reproducibility

Synonyms are reliability and repeatability. It is a measure of the consistency with which a question or a test will produce the same result on the same subject under similar conditions on successive occasions. A highly reproducible test must have low random error, although it may still have systematic error.

When reproducibility is evaluated by retesting subjects, it is usually defined as the ratio of the number of cases positive on both occasions to the number positive on at least one occasion. It can be assessed by:

Replication of tests: The results of a series of measurements by the same observer or by different observers using the same test on the same group of subjects (or set of specimens) under identical conditions are compared.

Comparison of test systems: The measurements are repeated using a different instrument or test system. Statistical analysis can be used to identify whether variation is attributable to the test system, intra-observer variation, inter-observer variation or subject variation. Similar methods can be applied to assessment of the reproducibility of questions, but there are problems because when the same question is repeated, the subject (and observer) may be conditioned by replies given on previous occasions. Additional procedures for assessing the reproducibility of questionnaires are:

• the use of check questions, that is questions which seek the same information though in a different form, e.g. age and date of birth;
• the random allocation of subjects to different interviewers and comparing results between groups.

Validity

Synonym is accuracy. This is a measure of the capacity of a test to give the true result. A valid test is one that correctly detects the presence or absence of a condition or places a subject correctly on a scale of measurement. For example, glycosuria as a test of the presence of diabetes has poor validity compared with a glucose tolerance test.

Validity has two components. In the case of a test which divides a population into two groups, validity is assessed by how well it picks up those with diseases (its *sensitivity*) and how well it rejects those without disease (its *specificity*). These two indices can be derived from a 2×2 table (Table 4.1) showing those with disease and those without according to the test result. In the perfectly valid test, c and b will be zero, that is there will be no false negatives and no false positives.

Table 4.1 Derivation of sensitivity and specificity of a test.

	With disease	Without disease	Total
Positive test	a True positive	b False positive	$-a + b$
Negative test	c False negative	d True negative	$c + d$
Total	$a + c$	$b + d$	T

$$\text{Sensitivity} = \frac{a}{(a + c)} = \frac{\text{True positive}}{\text{All with disease}}$$

$$\text{Specificity} = \frac{d}{(b + d)} = \frac{\text{True negative}}{\text{All without disease}}$$

Different methods are used to validate tests that give measurements on a scale (continuous variables) rather than assign people to a category. For example, an individual cannot be assigned within the categories diseased/not diseased on the basis of blood pressure because there is no agreed level of blood pressure which signifies the presence of disease. Continuous variables are validated by measuring the degree of concordance (agreement) between the results obtained by two different methods of measurement, or by relating observed values for measurements to certain criteria of outcome, e.g. ECG changes against the subsequent incidence of myocardial infarction.

Chapter 5
Cohort Studies

Introduction

Cohort studies involve the investigation of groups of people who have not manifest the disease at the time they are recruited for study. The selected study group is observed over a period of time in order to measure the frequency of occurrence of the disease amongst people exposed to the suspected causal agent compared with its frequency amongst individuals not exposed.

Types of cohort study

Two broad types of *cohort* can be used:
  groups with special personal characteristics;
  groups with special exposures.

Groups with special personal characteristics

Groups of individuals who have special characteristics unrelated either to their risk of exposure or to their risk of disease and who are easy to follow-up provide useful cohorts for the investigation of many diseases. Cohorts that have been studied because they are easy to identify and follow-up over long periods of time include, for example, those selected because they belong to a profession of which a register is constantly maintained (doctors, nurses, etc); individuals who are members of a particular insurance scheme; employees in industries with a low turnover of workers.

At the time of recruitment to the study, the investigator identifies the characteristics of the subjects by the use of questionnaires or the measurement of any number of biological variables. They are then followed-up until a sufficient proportion have reached a pre-defined end point (the development of the disease being investigated or death). During the follow-up period their exposures to suspected harmful agents are recorded.

Such cohorts can be used to estimate prevalence, incidence and risk in relation to a suspected causal agent without recruiting an additional comparison (control) group because the comparison group (those not exposed to the agent being investigated) is a sub-group of the cohort itself. This is called an *internal control* group.

Groups with special exposures

The other main type of cohort comprises groups of individuals who have all been exposed to the agent or the experience that is being investigated. This type of cohort requires the concurrent recruitment and study of an *external control* group. The control group must be drawn from a similar population to the exposed group in all respects other than exposure to the agent under investigation. The data on the control group must be the same and collected in the same way as that on the exposed group.

These two types of cohort can be equally valuable in epidemiological studies. The choice depends on the question being studied and the availability of suitable study populations.

Time at risk

In an ideal situation all members of a cohort (of either type) are recruited to a study at about the same time and followed-up for the same period of time. Sometimes it is not possible to recruit sufficient numbers to yield significant results in a short period, particularly if exposure to the agent being investigated is relatively rare. Moreover, in most studies some patients are lost to follow-up. Either situation will result in variations in the length of time for which the individual members of cohorts are observed. This will give rise to problems in the analysis of the data.

One way to handle variations in the periods during which individuals have been observed can be handled by using the total time at risk in each *group* as the denominator. It is calculated by summating the lengths of time each person in the group was exposed to risk or kept under observation for a particular outcome. It is expressed as the number of units of time at risk, e.g. 1 person-year = one individual at risk (or observed) for 1 year. An example is shown in Table 5.1.

However, caution must be exercised in the use of 'time at risk' as a denominator. It is only valid if the risk of developing the disease in an individual is not influenced by the period of exposure. In comparative studies of the efficacy of contraceptives it may be a legitimate procedure since it is unlikely that the risk of pregnancy after 1 year of exposure to oral contraceptives differs from the risk after 5 years of exposure or that the risk of pregnancy after 1 year's use of an IUD differs from that after 5 years of use. On the other hand, if there is reason to believe that the risk of a disease is affected by the length of time an individual is exposed to an agent the summation of the exposed time within a group will be misleading. For example in 1969 Pisciotta demonstrated that chlorpromazine can cause agranulocytosis in some people and that it usually occurs after 5–7 weeks of continuous exposure (Pisciotta A V. *JAMA* 1969; **208**: 1862). Thus patients who are exposed for less than 5 weeks are not 'at risk' since they would not have been exposed for a sufficient time for the reaction to occur, even

Table 5.1 The effectiveness of oral contraceptives expressed in terms of the number of unplanned pregnancies per hundred women-years of use.

Contraceptive used	Pregnancies per 100 women-years of use
Oral contraceptives	0.15
Diaphragm	2.40–5.00
IUD	2.00

though they might be susceptible. Patients exposed for over 7 weeks clearly have a greatly reduced risk of developing the dyscrasia since they have passed through the critical exposure period. If, in a study designed to assess the risk of agranulocytosis in patients exposed to chlorpromazine, the total number of treatment weeks is used as a denominator, it will give a distorted indication of the level of risk. In this case the definition of exposure must specify the time period during which the individual consumes the drug.

Advantages and disadvantages of cohort studies

Advantages

- The main advantage of the cohort study design is that it is possible to distinguish antecedent causes from associated factors in the aetiology of disease.
- In both types of cohort study the incidence of disease in exposed and non-exposed groups can be determined, allowing the calculation not only of absolute risk but also of relative and attributable risks (see p. 10).
- It is also possible to study several possible outcomes from exposure to the same hazard.
- Bias in controls is less of a problem than in case-control studies because the necessary comparison groups (exposed and non-exposed) are built into the study design from the start. Even so, it is important to bear in mind that the two groups may not be equally susceptible to the disease under study.
- Because the study is prospectively designed, it is possible to standardize methods, thereby reducing error due to observer, subject and technical variation (see p. 33).

Disadvantages

- It is still not possible to be absolutely sure that supposed aetiological factors really are causal. This requires experiments of a kind referred to in Chapter 3 which are rarely possible in human populations.
- Even with common diseases, large populations are usually required to obtain significant differences in incidence in exposed and non-exposed groups. Also, if the incubation period is prolonged, results may be greatly delayed. These factors tend to make cohort studies very expensive in resources.
- One of the major difficulties encountered in cohort studies is in the follow-up of all subjects. Migration and withdrawal of cooperation may bias the results. It is necessary, therefore, to build into the study design a system for obtaining basic information on the personal characteristics and outcome for those who cannot be followed up in detail for the full duration of the study. This allows comparisons to be made between subjects who are fully studied and those who are not. In this way serious selective bias may be detected and can be allowed for in the analysis and interpretation of the results.
- Finally, even though standard methods and diagnostic criteria are adopted, these may 'drift' over a prolonged follow-up period and results at the end may not be comparable with those obtained at the start.

Examples of cohort studies

Smoking and carcinoma of the bronchus amongst British doctors (Doll R, Hill A B. *Br Med J* 1964; **1**: 1399.)

The study of the effects of smoking amongst British doctors is a good example of a study based upon a cohort that was used because it was administratively easy to identify and follow-up. It involved the use of an 'internal control group'. In 1951 the research team sent a simple questionnaire to all of the 59 600 doctors whose names were on the British Medical Register at the time. The questionnaire enquired about their past and current smoking habits. Sixty-nine per cent of the male doctors and 60% of the female doctors who were contacted completed the questionnaire. The responding doctors were divided according to their past and current smoking habits and their subsequent mortality was recorded. A further questionnaire to obtain information on changes in smoking habits and other data was sent to the male doctors in 1957 and to the female doctors in 1960. The fact that all the individuals being studied were doctors on the British Medical Register aided follow-up considerably. Deaths of doctors are notified to the Medical Register, for reasons quite unconnected with the study, which enabled the investigators to follow-up a cohort many years after it was recruited with comparative ease. The first stage of the analysis was to divide the doctors into those exposed to the suspected harmful agent (smokers) and those not exposed (non-smokers). The mortality within the two groups was then compared.

The results of the study are well known and the conclusions of the investigators have had far-reaching consequences. An association between smoking and seven causes of death was found amongst the male doctors. The most pronounced was a linear correlation between the death rate from lung cancer and the number of cigarettes smoked (Fig. 5.1). The data also revealed that the risk of death from lung cancer fell substantially in those who gave up smoking, a benefit which increased with time (Fig. 5.2).

This study yielded two observations that could not have been made from descriptive studies alone. Firstly, the sequence of events was clearly identified, smoking was followed by lung cancer, and secondly a dose–response effect was demonstrated. Both of these findings weigh heavily in favour of the causal hypothesis. However, it should be remembered that the investigation was stimulated by the results of descriptive studies which showed a correlation between mortality from lung cancer and sales of cigarettes in England and Wales.

The problem with a cohort recruited in this way is that if it is used to study the effects of an agent or factor which is very rare, or if the disease is a rare consequence of exposure, then the size of the cohort has to be very large in order to yield sufficient numbers of cases to detect a significant difference between the risks in the exposed group and the non-exposed group.

Survivors of the Hiroshima and Nagasaki atomic explosions (Brill A B, Masanobu R R, Heyssel R M. *Ann Int Med* 1962; **56**: 590.)

The second type of cohort, one which is defined by the fact that the individual members have all been exposed to the same experience or agent, has the closest

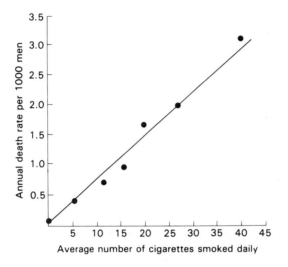

Fig. 5.1 Death rate from lung cancer standardized for age among men smoking daily numbers of cigarettes at the start of the inquiry (men smoking pipes or cigars as well as cigarettes, excluded). (From Doll R and Hill A B, 1964.)

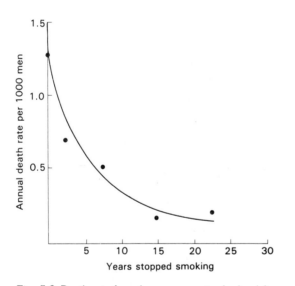

Fig. 5.2 Death rate from lung cancer, standardized for age and amount smoked, among men continuing to smoke cigarettes and men who had given up smoking for different periods (men who regularly smoked pipes or cigars as well as cigarettes excluded). (From Doll R and Hill A B, 1964.)

similarity to the laboratory experiment. There are many instances of cohorts that have been defined in this way. For example, the survivors of the atomic bomb explosions in Hiroshima and Nagasaki comprise a unique group of people who were exposed to high levels of ionizing radiation for a short time. In this group of people there was little difficulty in calculating the proportion who developed leukaemia after, say 10 years, i.e. the absolute risk of leukaemia. However, in order to establish whether the incidence of leukaemia in the cohort was more or less than in a group not so exposed, the relative risk of leukaemia, it was necessary to study a group of people who were similar to the exposed group in all respects except for their exposure to ionizing radiation. In one of the many studies of the survivors from Hiroshima and Nagasaki, the control group comprised individuals who were living in the same area but outside the radiation zone. The study showed that the incidence of confirmed leukaemia was between fifty and one hundred times greater in the exposed population than in the controls. Further investigations showed a clear relationship between the distance from the epicentre of the explosion and leukaemia incidence rates (Table 5.2), demonstrating a dose–response effect.

Table 5.2 Average incidence of confirmed leukaemia in residents of Hiroshima and Nagasaki (1947–1958) by city of exposure distance from epicentre.

Distance from epicentre (metres)	Incidence rate per 1 000 000 man-years at risk	
	Hiroshima	Nagasaki
0–999	1366	563
1000–1499	308	530
1500–1999	42	68
2000–9999	28	37

Regular fluoroscopy and risk of breast cancer (Boice J D, Monson R R. *J Nat Cancer Inst* 1977; **59**: 823.)

A cohort that experienced a different type of ionizing radiation is exemplified by the group of people who had large numbers of fluoroscopies in the 1940s and 1950s while being treated for pulmonary tuberculosis before the dangers of X-rays were fully appreciated. It has been shown that young women in the group that were irradiated had a higher than expected incidence of breast cancer. In this study the control group was all other women of the same age in the population, the great majority of whom, it may be assumed, were not exposed to radiation in this way (Table 5.3).

Social class differences in ischaemic heart disease in men (Pocock S J, Shaper A G, Cook D G, Phillips A N, Walker M. *Lancet* 1987; **ii**: 197.)

During 1979–1980, 7735 men aged 40–59 years were randomly selected from the 'lists' of persons registered with general practitioners in 24 towns in England, Scotland or Wales and were asked to participate in a long-term study. Seventy-eight per cent of those approached, agreed to cooperate. These men were asked to complete a questionnaire which included questions on occupation, smoking habits and indicators of heart disease. They were also examined by a research nurse. Ninety-nine per cent of the men were followed-up for an average of 6 years.

Table 5.3 Relative risk of breast cancer in women subjected to regular fluoroscopies at different ages (risk in general population = 1).

Age at first exposure (years)	Relative risk
<15	2.1
15–19	3.8
20–24	1.7
25–29	1.6
30–34	1.2
35–39	0.8
40 +	0.9

The data were analysed using a multiple logistic regression model in order to simultaneously adjust the incidence rates of major ischaemic heart disease events for smoking, systolic blood pressure, serum cholesterol, age and social class.

Of these men, 336 experienced major IHD events (defined as fatal IHD or myocardial infarction). The crude attack rates and the attack rates adjusted for the risk factors set out above are shown in Table 5.4.

This indicates that after taking account of the differences in smoking habits, systolic blood pressure, serum cholesterol and age between the social class groups, there remains an unexplained increase in incidence of major IHD events amongst men in manual occupations as compared to those in non-manual occupations.

Table 5.4 Attack rates of major IHD events during follow-up, before and after adjustment for social class differences in risk factors.

Social class	Number of IHD cases	Cases per 1000 per annum	
		Adjusted	Unadjusted
I	21	5.6 ⎱	7.4 ⎱
II	56	5.2 ⎰ 5.5	6.0 ⎰ 6.0
III Non-manual	27	6.0 ⎰	6.0 ⎰
III Manual	169	8.2 ⎱	7.7 ⎱
IV	36	7.4 ⎰ 7.9	7.3 ⎰ 7.5
V	11	5.6 ⎰	5.0 ⎰

Chapter 6
Case-control Studies

Introduction

Case-control studies are concerned with the analysis of events that occurred before the onset of the disease in the cases and before recruitment to the study. They are therefore sometimes called *retrospective studies*. They cannot answer all the same questions that can be explored with a cohort study. Often a case-control study is used for the preliminary investigation of an hypothesis, followed by a cohort study to explore and test the hypothesis more fully, as, for example, Doll and Hill did in their studies of the association between smoking and lung cancer (see p. 41). They involve comparing individuals who are identified because they are known to have the disease (cases) with individuals who do not have the disease being investigated (controls). The past histories and exposures to suspected harmful agents of cases and controls are ascertained either by direct questioning or by reference to their clinical or other records. The frequencies with which the same characteristics are found in the two groups are compared. The simplest comparisons are of the frequency rates of the antecedent factors between groups. Thereafter it may be profitable to use more complex statistical techniques that take account of more than one variable at a time. A greater frequency of a factor under investigation in the diseased group lends support to an aetiological hypothesis, but it will not necessarily prove a causal hypothesis. This is because the sequence of events is not always clear. For example, if men with coronary heart disease are found to follow a sedentary occupation more often than controls, it is not clear whether lack of exercise predisposes to heart disease or whether those with incipient cardiac problems choose less physically demanding jobs.

Selection of cases

The value of a case-control study is profoundly influenced by the ways in which both the cases and the controls are selected. Ideally all the cases of the disease in a defined population should be included in the investigation. In practice it is rarely necessary to do this in order to reach sensible and valid conclusions. Furthermore it is rarely feasible to be so comprehensive in recruitment. Most studies are implicitly or explicitly concerned with a sample of cases, usually identified by some form of cluster sampling technique (see p. 32). The 'cluster' used will depend upon the disease that is being investigated and the availability and accessibility of information about patients who are affected by the disease. Sources that are commonly used to identify cases include hospital in-patients, patients attending hospital out-patient departments or their general practitioner, patients who are on disease registers such as cancer registers, and death certificates. Whatever the source that is used, it is important to establish that all persons with the disease have an equal chance of appearing at that source if it is intended to extrapolate the findings of the study beyond the circumstances in which it was undertaken.

These principles can be illustrated by considering the selection of cases for a study of the risk factors associated with carcinoma of the breast. It is reasonable to recruit the cases from amongst women being treated in hospital for the first time for breast cancer, as there is a high probability that all cases of breast cancer will receive hospital treatment or hospital care before they die and without treatment the disease is nearly always fatal. By contrast, the identification of cases for a study of peptic ulcer is more difficult. Not all people with peptic ulceration seek medical help for their condition. The identification of cases at a source of medical care may introduce bias into the investigation because the factors that lead an individual to seek attention are not necessarily related either to the severity of the disease or its symptoms. In effect patients who seek medical attention for a peptic ulcer, whether at hospital or in general practice, are not a random sample of individuals affected with a peptic ulcer. The more specialized the source of these patients, e.g. gastroenterology in-patients, the more selective is the group and consequently general conclusions from the results of the study become less secure. In situations such as this it is often necessary to conduct a prevalence survey in a general population (see p. 29) in order to identify cases for inclusion in a study.

Once the appropriate source of patients for study has been identified, the 'cluster', the same principles of sampling from the cluster can be applied as have been explained in Chapter 4.

Selection of controls

Control subjects are essential in order to establish the frequency with which the suspected causal agents or determinants occur in people who do not have the disease under investigation. Controls should be a random sample of the population from which the cases were recruited. Once selected, controls should neither be discarded nor replaced for any reason other than that they fail to meet the selection criteria, e.g. they were mistakenly drawn from another population.

The similarity between controls and cases can be ensured by selecting controls individually to match cases by specific criteria, e.g. age, sex, and any other variable which may affect the risk of exposure to an agent or risk of contracting disease but which is not one of the variables under study. These are called *matched pairs*. The limitation of using this method of selection is that the effects of the characteristics which form the basis of the matching cannot be assessed. Alternatively matching may be on a group basis, i.e. selection of controls at random from a sample of the parent population from which the cases were drawn. Sometimes, in order to increase statistical sensitivity in the analysis of the results, more than one control is selected for each case, particularly if the number of cases is small. Data must be obtained and observations made in a precisely similar manner for controls as for cases.

It is important to note that the error or bias in the selection of controls will have exactly the same effect on the outcome of the study as bias in the selection of cases. In case-control studies (and in cohort studies that involve selection of external controls) as much attention must be given to the identification of and collection of data from the control subjects as is given to the cases.

Control subjects can be recruited from the following list of examples.

• Persons working in the same factory or attending the same school or living in the same locality as cases.

• Routine registers such as birth registers, electoral rolls, payrolls, school rolls or general practice lists. Each of these has its own selective bias which must be recognized in making a choice.

• Hospital patients, either all attenders or, more usually, those with conditions belived to be unrelated to the factors under study. The main limitation of using hospital patients as controls in any study is that, even though they may not have the disease being investigated, they are unlikely to be a random sample of the general population from which the cases are drawn. For example, even though a hospital patient does not have the disease under investigation he or she may have another disease whose presence could have affected exposure to the causal agent of the disease under investigation. Moreover people who live in poor social environments are more likely to be admitted to hospital than those who live in better circumstances and their use as controls will introduce a social class bias.

• Relatives and spouses. These have the advantage of accessibility and willingness to cooperate, ease of location and of sharing the same environmental conditions. Obviously they are unsuitable where genetic or home environment factors are under study. It is also unlikely that such a selection process will result in the same sex ratio as the cases unless the occurrence of the disease is unrelated to sex.

• Recently control subjects for some case-control studies have been identified through random digit dialling using telephone exchanges serving the areas in which the cases are resident. Using this method, controls that fail to meet basic recruitment criteria are discarded after a few key questions and the remainder are included in the investigation.

Risk in cohort and case-control studies

Cohort studies are designed to provide the data needed to calculate incidence rates of the disease amongst individuals exposed to the suspected causal agent and those not exposed. By contrast, case-control studies only provide the data from which the rate of exposure to suspected harmful agents in diseased and non-diseased individuals can be calculated. This means that neither the absolute nor the relative or attributable risk resulting from exposure can be calculated. The difficulty is shown schematically in Tables 6.1 and 6.2.

In a cohort study the subjects studied are all those exposed $(A + C)$ and all those not exposed $(B + D)$ to the suspected causal agent (Table 6.1). The subjects subsequently reveal themselves as diseased or non-diseased within these categories. There is, therefore, no difficulty in calculating the disease rate in the exposed patients $[A/(A + C)]$ and those not exposed $[B/(B + D)]$. The subsequent calculation of relative risk (RR) and attributable risk (AR) presents no problem:

$$RR = \frac{A}{A+C} \bigg/ \frac{B}{B+D}$$

$$AR = \frac{A}{A+C} - \frac{B}{B+D}$$

The subjects in a case-control study are identified either because they have the disease (the cases) or because they do not have the disease (the controls) that is being investigated. They are subsequently sub-divided into 'exposed' and 'not exposed' sub-groups (Table 6.2). It is not possible to derive the total numbers of cases in the population who were exposed and not exposed because a case-control study is not based upon a known proportion of the population. Consequently neither the incidence rate in the population as a whole nor the incidence rate amongst the people exposed to the suspected harmful agent can be derived. It follows from this that risk cannot be calculated directly. An approximation of the relative risk can be derived from case-control data. This approximation although usually referred to as the relative risk is more correctly termed the *odds ratio* (OR).

Table 6.1 Information available in cohort studies.

	Disease present	Disease absent	Total
Exposed to suspected cause	A	C	$A+C$
Not exposed to suspected cause	B	D	$B+D$

Table 6.2 Division of subjects in a case-control study.

	Diseased	Not diseased
Suspected cause present	a	c
Suspected cause absent	b	d
Total	$a+b$	$c+d$

Using the notation in Table 6.1 the true relative risk is:

$$\frac{A \times (B+D)}{B \times (A+C)}$$

In the case of most diseases, the proportion of the population who are affected, whether or not they are exposed to the suspected causal agent is small. Thus A is small in relation to C; likewise B is small in relation to D. It follows that D will approximate to $(B+D)$ and C will approximate to $(A+C)$. The approximation to the relative risk OR then becomes:

$$\frac{A \times D}{B \times C} = \frac{a \times d}{b \times c}$$

This approximation to relative risk is used in all case-control studies but it is only valid if the incidence of the disease is low.

It is not possible in most circumstances to calculate attributable risk from a case-control study.

Adjusting for confounding variables

There are two ways of taking account of confounding variables:

1   Analysis of sub-sets of the data to adjust for the confounding variable.

This can be illustrated by considering a study of the effect of age of first birth on the risk of carcinoma of the breast. Women who have their first child whilst young tend to have more children than women whose first child is born late in their reproductive life. It follows that if there is a statistical association between age of first birth and the risk of breast cancer it is likely that there will also be an association between family size and risk of breast cancer. The two effects can be separated by restricting the analysis to women who have had only one child (thereby separating out the effects of parity) and calculating the risk according to age of first pregnancy. Or the analysis can be restricted to women who had their first child at a given age and calculating the risks according to parity. The disadvantage of this technique is that it means that not all the data can be used in the critical analyses.

2   Use of a logistic regression technique to adjust the relative risk for the effect of confounding variables.

The advent of accessible and powerful computing has made it possible to use more sophisticated mathematical techniques to analyse data from epidemiological studies. The calculation of an adjusted relative risk using logistic regression is one such application. An advantage of this technique is that it allows simultaneous adjustment for the effects of more than one confounding variable. Similar methods are used to adjust for the effects of confounding variables in cohort studies. A discussion of the mathematics of this method is beyond the scope of this text; it is considered by Armitage and Berry (see Appendix).

Effects of high incidence of exposure

Essentially the success of a case-control study is dependent upon there being a difference between the proportion of cases exposed to the suspect agent and the number of controls so exposed. If the incidence of exposure is very high it may be impossible to demonstrate such a difference. Consider an extreme example of a case-control study designed to identify the possible causal agents of carcinoma of the bronchus which is conducted in a population where the prevalence of cigarette smoking over the age of 15 years is 100%. In such a situation there can be no difference between the proportion of cases and controls exposed to cigarettes. It follows that smoking cannot be revealed as a risk factor. It does not follow that no risk factors will be revealed by such a study, but those identified may be associated rather than causal and the principal cause will be missed.

Advantages and disadvantages of case-control studies

Advantages

Despite the approximations that have to be made in the analysis of case-control studies, they do have some important advantages over cohort studies.

• By concentrating effort on the identification of affected individuals and recruiting controls from the unaffected population the number of subjects required to obtain significant results is kept to a minimum.

• Results can be obtained relatively quickly because the investigation does not have to wait for the disease to develop as it does in cohort studies. This means that it is a relatively inexpensive type of study.

Disadvantages

• Case-control studies generally rely upon retrospective data collection and data of this type have their own inherent problems. The ability of individuals to recall past events tends to be unreliable due to a tendency for memory to be selective. Records of past events may be incomplete in respect of variables that are deemed important by investigators. The ways in which observations and measurements are made are not usually standardized and this gives rise to uncertainty regarding their validity.

• Because the data are collected after the event (retrospectively) it is difficult to be sure whether a demonstrable correlation is causal or not. Thus, the finding that a history of cigarette smoking is common amongst individuals with lung cancer does not prove that the former preceded and caused the latter. Alternative explanations are that people who choose to smoke are also constitutionally predisposed to lung cancer or are exposed to another noxious agent more often than are non-smokers. This problem is less conspicuous when dealing with highly specific agents such as micro-organisms or in situations where the time between exposure and onset of symptoms is short.

• There are sometimes difficulties in selecting and recruiting appropriate controls. This is important because the value of the results obtained from a case-control study is as dependent upon the proper selection of 'controls' as it is on the identification of affected individuals.

• Because case-control studies are not based on defined populations the incidence of the disease within that population cannot be calculated from the study.

Examples of case-control studies

Sexual activity, contraceptive method, genital infections and cervical cancer

(Slattery M, Overall J C, Abbott T M et al. Am J Epidemiol 1989: **130**; 248–258.)

It has been suggested that cervical cancer is a sexually transmitted disease. Between 1984 and 1987 a case-control study was carried out in Utah (USA) where a high proportion of the population are active members of the Church of Jesus Christ of Latter Day Saints (Mormons). The study was designed to explore the relationship between cervical cancer and sexual activity, the use of barrier methods of contraception and certain types of genital infection. The subjects were women aged 20–59 years, newly diagnosed with cervical cancer. Controls were identified by use of a random digit dialling telephone sampling technique. They were matched to cases by 5-year age intervals and county of residence. Interviews were completed for 266 women with histologically confirmed carcinoma *in situ* or invasive squamous cell cervical cancer and for 408 matched controls.

After adjustment for age, education, church attendance and cigarette smoking, by means of multiple logistic regression models, several significant risk factors were identified. These included multiple sex partners, current mate having multiple sex partners, reported trichomonas infection and serological evidence of herpes virus type 2 infection (Table 6.3). It should be noted that there is a pronounced gradient of risk relating to increased numbers of partners and increased numbers of partners of the mate of the woman.

A protective effect was noted from use of foam or jelly as a contraceptive method (OR = 0.44), from the use of diaphragms (OR = 0.67) or condoms in women who reported more than one sex partner (OR = 0.53). These data lend support to the hypothesis that cervical cancer is transmitted sexually.

Whooping cough vaccine and severe neurological illness (Miller D L, Ross E M, Alderslade R, Bellman M H, Rawson N S B. *Br Med J* 1981; **282**: 1595.)

In 1975 widespread public alarm was created by the suggestion that whooping

Table 6.3 Risk factors and cervical cancer.

Risk factor	Numbers		Odds ratio	
	Cases	Controls	Crude	Adjusted
Number of sex partners of woman				
<2	25	210	1.00	1.00
2–3	54	73	6.21	3.43
4–5	47	53	7.44	3.59
6–10	57	39	12.27	5.51
>10	69	28	20.70	8.99
Number of sex partners of mate				
1	24	198	1.00	1.00
2–3	42	78	4.44	2.72
4–5	38	39	8.03	4.99
6–10	45	22	16.87	7.98
>10	49	23	17.57	8.62
Trichomonas infections	53	21	4.61	2.10
Herpes type 2 (neutralization index >100)	12	6	6.57	2.70

cough vaccine might cause severe encephalopathic illnesses followed by permanent brain damage in a small but significant number of children. It would have been impractical and unethical to conduct a large scale randomized control trial to test the validity of this suggestion. Therefore a case-control study was set up which aimed to identify all children admitted to hospitals in Britain with serious acute neurological illnesses of the types which it was suggested could be caused by the vaccine and lead to permanent brain damage. For each case child reported, two control children, matched for age and sex, were selected from those living in the same local area. The past histories of possible predisposing or aetiological factors were obtained for both case and control children in identical manners. Of the first 1000 cases notified, 35 (3.5%) had received pertussis vaccine within 7 days before becoming ill, compared with 34 (1.7%) of 1955 control children, a significant excess of observed over expected (OR = 2.4). Thus the study showed that there is a small but definite risk attached to whooping cough vaccine, though the risk was much smaller than some workers had suggested from totally uncontrolled series of cases.

Smoking and lung cancer (Doll R, Hill A B. *Br Med J* 1950; **ii**: 739.)

In 1950, Doll and Hill undertook a case-control study to 'determine whether patients with carcinoma of the lung differed materially from other persons in respect of their smoking habits or in some other way. . .'. They arranged for 20 hospitals in London to notify them of all patients admitted with cancer of the lung. For patients admitted with cancer of the lung a 'control' patient without this form of cancer was selected; the control was of the same sex, within the same 5-year age group and in the same hospital at or about the same time as the case.

Altogether 649 men and 60 women with carcinoma of the lung and the same number of control subjects were interviewed. Among those with lung cancer 0.3% of men and 31.7% of women were non-smokers compared with 4.2% of men and 53.3% of women among controls. Patients who had cancer of the lung were shown to fall predominantly in the heavier-smoking categories (Fig. 6.1). It seemed unlikely that these results could be accounted for by any bias in the method and it was concluded that smoking was probably an important factor in the aetiology of carcinoma of the lung. However, it required a cohort study (see p. 41) to confirm the hypothesis.

Perinatal deaths and maternal occupation (Clarke M, Mason E S. *Br Med J* 1985; **290**: 1235–7.)

Reproductive hazards are thought to exist in many industries. In order to explore this problem, a case-control study of perinatal death occurring in Leicestershire was carried out between 1976 and 1982. Case notes were reviewed and the mothers were interviewed in all 1187 cases of perinatal death during this period. The control for each case was selected as the next live birth occurring at the place, or intended place of delivery. All maternal and paternal occupations and industries were recorded at the interview with the mother. A total of 671

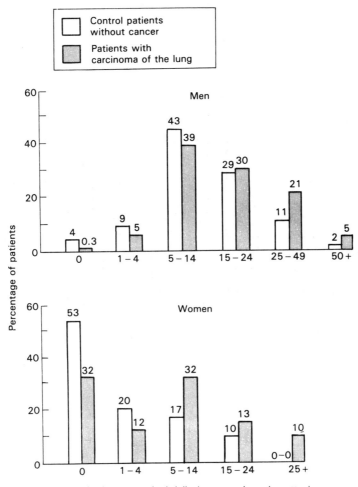

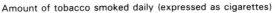

Amount of tobacco smoked daily (expressed as cigarettes)

Fig. 6.1 Percentage of patients smoking different amounts of tobacco daily. (From Doll R, Hill A B. *Br Med J* 1950: **2**: 739.)

mothers were employed outside the home at some time during pregnancy. An analysis of maternal occupations showed that the OR for the risk of perinatal death was exceptionally high in women employed in the leather industry (OR = 2.1 after adjustment for social class). A similar excess was found in all towns within the county where shoe manufacture took place. No other risk factor was found to account for this observation. Possible hazards appeared to be the leather or adhesives used or both. Further studies will be required to identify the specific hazardous exposure in these women.

Chapter 7
Intervention Studies

Introduction

Descriptive and analytic studies are used to develop and test hypotheses about the possible causes and determinants of disease. The results may suggest methods of prevention or treatment which then need to be formally evaluated. Intervention studies are most often used for this purpose and are commonly called *clinical trials*. They are essentially experimental studies in which the efficacy and safety of medical management of disease is evaluated by comparing the outcome of the intervention in test and control groups. The intervention under test is most often a new preventive or treatment regime, but the method can also be used to compare different regimes and to evaluate the effectiveness and efficiency of different forms of service provision. Experimental studies in which the incidence of a disease in those deliberately exposed to a suspected causal agent, or protected from it, is compared with that in controls can also be of value and provide the most convincing evidence of cause. However, for practical and ethical reasons this approach is rarely adopted except in animal studies.

Methods in clinical trials

The methodologies of preventive and therapeutic trials have some similarities to those used in cohort study. The basis of a clinical trial is the random allocation of individuals in a population to 'test' and 'control' groups. The intervention measure under trial is applied to the test group but not to the control group and the effect is assessed in terms of a defined *outcome* in both groups. The particular form of intervention whose effects are being tested is called the *independent variable*, while the outcome being measured is called the *dependent variable*. The selection of the study population should be governed by the following considerations:

• The population under study should be representative of the population in which it is intended to apply the intervention being tested (this is called the *reference population*).

• It is important to choose a stable population in which there are unlikely to be heavy losses during the follow-up period and whose cooperation is reasonably assured. Volunteers are usually not acceptable since they tend to differ from non-volunteers in important respects, such as motivation and past history of illness.

• The likely frequency of the outcome being measured should be known since this critically affects the required sample size. It is usually convenient to choose a group with a high incidence of the outcome being investigated in order to economize on numbers.

- The population should be readily accessible. Trials are often most conveniently conducted in patients attending general practice or hospital, in residential institutions, factories, hospital patients, the armed forces, etc, even though they may not fairly represent the general population in all respects.

Allocation to test and control groups

In principle the allocation of patients to test and control groups should be random, hence the term sometimes applied to clinical trials, *randomized controlled trials* (RCT). The aim is to ensure that those treated and those untreated are exactly similar in all respects prior to intervention. This is necessary to guard against the possibility that some factor other than the intervention could account for differences in outcome in the two groups.

Individual allocation

The allocation of individuals to test or control groups can be by day of birth, registration number or other suitable procedure. This is the usual method adopted in clinical trials. Alternate allocation to test and control is to be avoided, as it may enable the patient or the person who assesses the outcome, to guess the group to which the patient has been allocated.

Cluster allocation

For practical reasons, allocation is sometimes made of whole groups or communities. This is because, e.g. in trials of a vaccine, the spread of infection may be inhibited in unvaccinated persons if a proportion of the population is protected, thereby obscuring the benefit derived from vaccination. Similarly in recent trials of preventive advice against coronary heart disease, the test and control groups were workers in randomly allocated factories, in order to minimize 'contamination' of the control group with advice offered to the intervention group.

Stratified allocation

Where the population is relatively small and non-homogeneous, random selection within specified sub-groups, e.g. age groups, may be desirable to ensure similarity in relevent characteristics between test and control groups.

No allocation

Sometimes random allocation of treatment would not be ethical, e.g. a trial of a new type of measles vaccine in children. In this case the comparison must be with past experience or that in other populations. It is difficult in such cases to measure the extent of any benefit with confidence.

Since willingness to cooperate may not be randomly distributed in the population, allocation should be deferred until agreement to participate has been obtained.

To avoid bias in reporting illnesses and other possible behavioral differences, subjects should not know to which group they have been allocated. In drug and vaccine trials this often entails the use of a placebo treatment for controls which must be presented in an identical form to the active treatment. In the case of some procedures, e.g. provision of different types of service, blind allocation is not possible. A trial in which neither the subject nor the persons assessing outcome know whether the subject is receiving active treatment or not (or which of two different treatments is being given) is called a *double-blind trial*.

Outcome (dependent variable)

The outcome to be assessed must be specified in advance. It should be expressed in terms of advantage to the patient or to the community, e.g. reduced incidence or severity of disease or cost to the health service. Assessment criteria should be clearly defined, consistently applied and reliably recorded in order to minimize bias in the measurement of outcome. Misclassified cases in either group will reduce the size of difference between the incidence of disease in test and control groups and thus give a spuriously reduced apparent benefit from the treatment. The assessment of outcome should always include the frequency of adverse effects of interventions as well as their benefits.

Follow-up

Procedures for the follow-up of subjects in both test and control groups should give attention to the following:
- The data collected must be obtained and recorded in a standard manner.
- The method used should be simple and should be sufficiently sensitive to reliably detect relevant events in members of the study population.
- Follow-up must be equally rigorous in both test and control groups
- Follow-up must start from the time of allocation and continue for long enough to evaluate fully the outcome in all subjects.
- Cooperation must be maintained at the highest possible level and losses from the study population for any reasons minimized.

Analysis

The *efficacy* of an intervention is usually measured as the proportion of the expected incidence which is prevented by the intervention expressed as a percentage, i.e.

$$\frac{[\text{expected incidence (controls)} - \text{intervention incidence (test)}] \times 100}{\text{expected incidence}}$$

For example, in a vaccine trial:
incidence in vaccinated children = 5 per thousand;
incidence in unvaccinated children = 50 per thousand.

$$\text{Efficacy} = \frac{50 - 5}{50} = \frac{45}{50} = 90\%$$

Sequential analysis

Sometimes, when a result is required urgently or when the anticipated benefits are high or the possible adverse effects are serious the results are analysed sequentially. This technique involves continuous data analysis and allows the trial to be stopped immediately a significantly beneficial or adverse effect has been demonstrated or when the results fail to reach a previously defined level of significance.

Ethical considerations

The ethical questions that arise in the planning and conduct of RCTs include:
- what are the possible risks of treatment and of failure to treat?
- Is it right to expose some people to possible harm from untested treatment or to withhold from others a possibly beneficial treatment?
- Is it right to introduce a new treatment into use without first assessing its safety and benefits by a properly conducted trial?
- To what extend should a trial be explained to the patients participating?
- How can the welfare and safety of participants be safeguarded while preserving the principle of 'blind' assessment?

In general it is best to carry out a trial before the new treatment is accepted into routine practice. Usually potent new drugs and vaccines are in short supply initially and it is impossible to offer them to everyone. At this stage random allocation of patients in a properly conducted trial may be as fair a means of selection as any and full advantage should be taken of the opportunity. Where omission of active treatment or giving a placebo may be dangerous, the controls are often given conventional treatment. In this case the aim is to measure the additional advantage from the new treatment.

The Medical Research Council (MRC), the World Health Organization (WHO) and others have issued guidelines for resolving some of the ethical problems of clinical trials. Health districts and research institutions now have 'Ethical Committees' with both broad professional and lay representation. These offer research workers the benefit of advice from a group of uncommitted individuals who can review the protocol dispassionately, though final responsibility must always rest with the scientist doing the work.

Examples of intervention studies

MRC trial of treatment of mild hypertension (Medical Research Council Working Party *Br Med J* 1985; **291**: 97–104)

It has long been known that people with high blood pressure have an increased risk of stroke and other cardiovascular events and that treatment is effective in reducing the incidence of these conditions in severe hypertension. However, the value of treating mild hypertension compared with disadvantages of long-term therapy in otherwise healthy people was less certain. A randomized control trial of treatment in such cases was therefore carried out by MRC. Even though hypertension and cardiovascular complications are relatively common conditions, it was calculated that this would require a very large scale trial in order to obtain a statistically significant result. Subjects for the trial were found by screening blood pressure measurements in 515 000 persons aged 35–64 years selected from the age–sex register of 176 general practices in England, Scotland and Wales.

In this way 17 354 patients with a diastolic pressure in the range 90–109 mmHg and systolic pressure below 200 mmHg were identified. Patients were randomly allocated to one of four groups, two of which were treated with different hypotensive drugs and two with placebo tablets which looked identical to the active drug tablets. Randomization was stratified by age and sex. The target level of blood pressure was below 90 mmHg to be reached within 6 months of entry. The study was single blind only—that is the doctor knew the treatment group to which the patients were allocated, but the patients did not. This was to enable the general practitioner to adjust drug dosage in those on active treatment if necessary to achieve the target level of blood pressure. All other management was the same in both treatment and placebo groups. Recruiting took place over 9 years and the data were analysed sequentially every 6 months in order to test whether any significant differences were emerging. In the end, 85 572 patient-years of observation accrued. There was a very significant reduction in the incidence of stroke in the treated group, but no difference in the rates of coronary events (Table 7.1). Overall incidence of cardiovascular events was reduced, but mortality from these and all causes was not. It was concluded that if 850 mildly hypertensive patients are given treatment for a year, about one stroke will be prevented. On the other hand, this would subject a substantial percentage of patients to chronic side effects, most but not all of which would be minor.

Prevention of rickets in Asian children: assessment of the Glasgow campaign
(Dunnigan M G, Glekin B M, Henderson J B et al. Br Med J 1985; **291**: 239–242.)

There have been many reports of vitamin D deficiency leading to rickets in infants and school children and osteomalacia in women among the British Asian community. Theoretically this would be easily remedied. The treatment is clear cut and no trial of the efficacy of vitamin D is needed. The acceptability of a prophylactic programme and its effectiveness in reducing the prevalence of rickets, however, needed to be assessed. Random allocation of individuals to treatment and control group would be inappropriate and unethical and, in such circumstances, though less than ideal, a *before* and *after* intervention assessment is often used. This study reported on the results of a campaign to promote the use of vitamin D supplementation in Glasgow. In a pre-campaign survey blood

Table 7.1 Mild hypertension: main events in treatment and control groups.

Event	Active treatment		Placebo		Percentage difference
	Number	Rate	Number	Rate	
Stroke	60	1.4	109	2.6	45
Coronary events	222	5.4	234	5.5	6
All cardiovascular events	286	6.7	352	8.2	19
All cardiovascular deaths	134	3.1	139	3.3	4
Non-cardiovascular deaths	114	2.7	114	2.7	0

samples were obtained from 189 children aged 5–17 years and those with biochemical evidence of rickets had an X-ray examination of the knees. In post-campaign surveys 2 and 3 years later, 255 children were similarly examined. On both occasions the children were asked about their frequency of consumption of vitamin D supplements (in younger children this was checked with mothers). The results showed a striking reduction in the prevalence of rickets in children who took regular or even intermittent vitamin D supplements, and the number of hospital discharges of Asian children with rickets in Glasgow declined rapidly after the start of the campaign.

Clearly the decline in rickets could have been due to factors other than the official vitamin D supplement campaign, for example, increasing adoption of a Western diet and lifestyle. However, the time and place reduction in rickets prevalence, backed by objective measures, lends support to an assessment of the effectiveness of the campaign.

A randomized controlled trial of anti-smoking advice: 10-year results (Rose G, Hamilton P J S, Colwell L, Shipley M J. *J Epidemiol Community Health* 1982; **36**: 102–108.)

Many studies have shown that the mortality and morbidity of ex-smokers is less than that of those who continue to smoke. On this basis smokers are confidently advised to give up smoking in the expectation that their health and prognosis will improve. However, ex-smokers are not a random sample of former smokers and their reasons for giving up may be related to other factors which influence their risk of developing smoking related diseases. Nor is it certain how effective anti-smoking advice is in influencing smoking behaviour. Therefore, in 1968 the authors set up a randomized control trial of anti-smoking advice in 1445 male smokers, aged 40–59 years, at high risk of developing cardiovascular disease. They were allocated at random to an 'intervention' group who were given individual advice on the relation of smoking to health and challenged to consider their situation. Those who declared a wish to stop smoking were given support and encouragement for an average of four or five visits over 12 months. The 'control' group were given no specific advice. All subjects completed a questionnaire 1, 3 and 9 years later. Deaths in the group were monitored. After 1 year the reported cigarette consumption in the intervention group was one-quarter of that in the control group and over 10 years the net reported reduction averaged 53%. The intervention group experienced fewer respiratory symptoms and less loss of ventilatory function. Their mortality from coronary heart disease was 18% lower than controls, and for lung cancer it was 23% lower. Unfortunately deaths from other cancers were higher than in controls, but this appeared to be a chance finding. It was concluded that the policy of encouraging smokers to give up the habit was worthwhile and should not be changed.

Chapter 8
Health Information and Information Systems

Introduction

Health is an elusive concept. The WHO has defined it as 'a state of complete physical, mental and social wellbeing'. It is, however, difficult if not impossible to use this definition to measure the health of populations in any categorical sense. Its principal limitation is that an individual's sense of 'wellbeing' is intimately related to that person's expectations from life; these are difficult to measure objectively. Therefore, in order to measure and compare the health of populations there are few alternatives other than to make use of indices of death and disease, despite the fact that these are the antithesis of health. The calculation of death rates and disease rates requires both numerator data (about the events being studied (death and disease)) and denominator data (about the populations in which the events take place).

This chapter is concerned with routinely collected data used in the measurement of health, mainly from official sources, and with the principles of information systems.

Census data

Most developed countries undertake regular and detailed censuses of their populations in order to provide information to assist in social and fiscal planning. Although there is evidence that many of the ancient empires, e.g. Babylon and Egypt, undertook occasional quite sophisticated censuses, it was the Romans who introduced it as a regular administrative exercise. They did this primarily for taxation assessment purposes. Perhaps the most famous Roman census was the one which took the parents of Christ to Bethlehem at the time of his birth. After the fall of the Roman Empire the regular counting of populations ceased. In England the first post-Roman attempt to enumerate the population resulted in the compilation of the Domesday Book in the eleventh century. In common with most of their predecessors the administrators at that time were concerned to identify families rather than individuals, and even families of different status were recorded differently. From the material that survives it is not possible to derive a precise figure of the population at that time.

The modern system of censuses was introduced in Europe during the late eighteenth and early nineteenth centuries. In England and Wales the first complete census was undertaken at the behest of Parliament in 1801. Since then there has been a full census every 10 years, with the exception of 1941. In recent years 10% sample censuses have been undertaken, midway between the full decennial censuses. The census is conducted by the Office of Population Censuses and Surveys (OPCS), a government department. Each census is

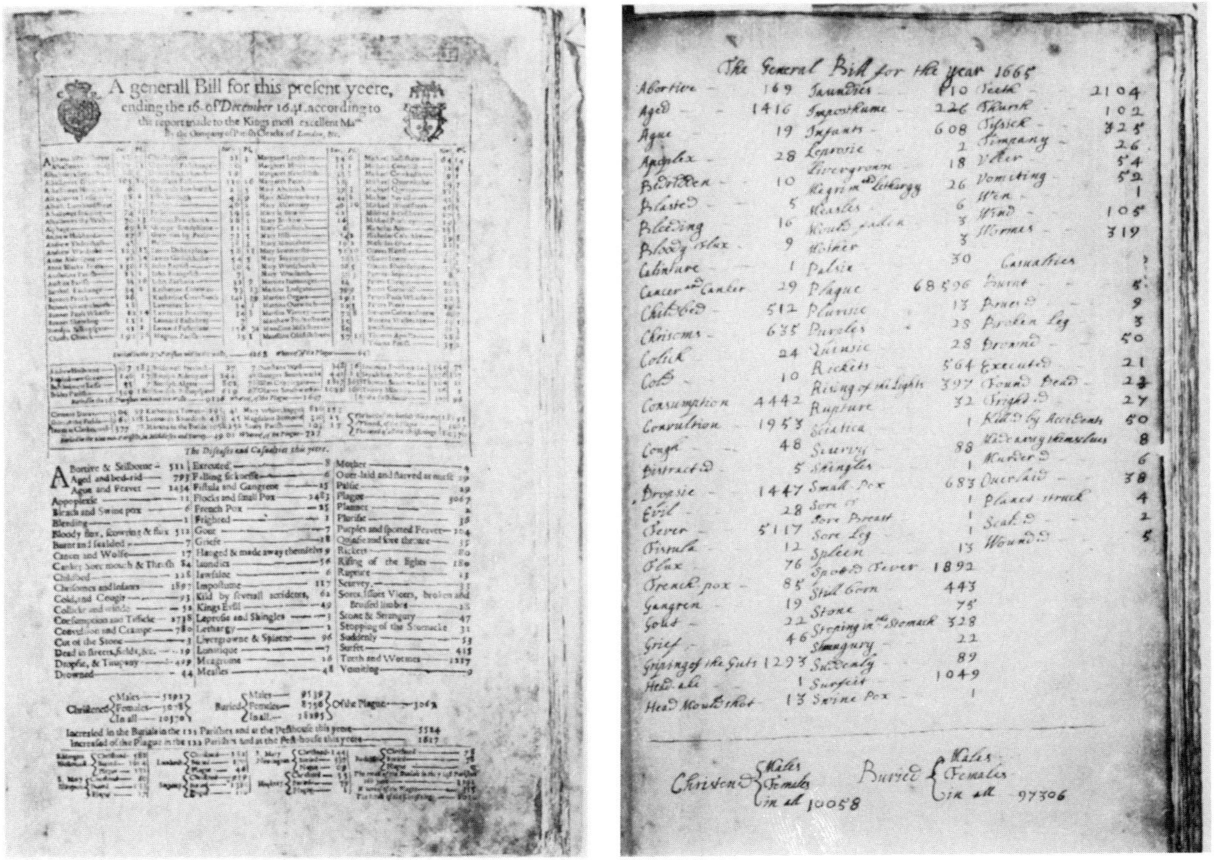

Fig. 8.1 The General Bills of Mortality 1641 and 1665.

undertaken only with the specific authority of Parliament. Any individual who refuses to cooperate is liable to prosecution.

The precise information that is collected varies from census to census but it invariably includes age, sex, marital condition, place of birth, occupation, number of children, usual place of residence and duration of present residence. In addition the head of the household has to furnish details of the residence including its type, tenure, accommodation and facilities. In recent years it has been the practice to ask for additional information from a sample of the population. All the information relating to individuals is confidential, even within government departments.

Before census day, officials deliver the appropriate census form to each household and institution in the country. They are collected by the same official after census day, who is available to help householders with any problems they encounter. The data on the forms are now analysed centrally by computer. In the past, tabulations of census data have been published as books, some of the more detailed information only after a delay of several years because of the time required for analysis and printing. The 1981 census was published both as books and as computer-readable magnetic tape. Despite some problems arising from concealment or misreporting of census information, and slight under recording because some people are not at a formal address on census night, modern censuses are regarded as being generally very accurate.

Estimates of population between censuses

The size and demographic characteristics of the population in non-census years is estimated by deducting deaths and emigrants from numbers recorded in the census and adding births and immigrants. At the same time the age distribution of the people remaining is adjusted. These are known as *inter-censal estimates*. Unfortunately errors occur and they are compounded by the passage of time. The principle sources of error in the inter-censal estimates arise through inadequate recording of immigration and emigration both in numbers and in respect of age and sex. Furthermore there is no system for ascertaining the amount of internal migration (changes of residence within the country). Thus the greater the time that has elapsed since a census, the less the precision of the estimate, especially estimates relating to small areas within the country. After a census the figures for years since the last census are recalculated, taking account of the information provided by the new census. These are called *post-censal estimates*.

Population projections

For planning purposes it is often essential to have some idea of the likely size and composition of the population in years to come. The essential difference between population estimates and population projections is that an *estimate* is based on knowledge of the births, deaths and migration that have happened, and a *projection* is based upon what is thought likely to happen. Therefore assumptions have to be made about trends in mortality, birth rates and migration. These are arrived at by extrapolating past trends. Unforeseen changes in, for example fertility, can invalidate the projections.

Vital events

General

Since the early nineteenth century, there has been a statutory requirement for all births, deaths and marriages in Britain to be registered. Before the Births, Marriages and Deaths Act (1839) most of the records that existed were kept by the ecclesiastical authorities. Since the vast majority of the population at that time were baptized in infancy, the numbers of baptisms recorded in the parish registers can be used as proxy indicators of the numbers of live births. There was no information on still births. As most marriages were in church, marriage rates also can be computed from the parish records. Likewise most of the population received Christian burials and therefore the fact of death was usually recorded. However, the presumed cause of death was of little interest to the ecclesiastical authorities and was not routinely noted. In the seventeenth century 'Bills of Mortality' were published for some large towns and cities. The best known are those compiled by John Graunt (Fig. 8.1). The cause of death was arrived at by paying lay 'searchers', normally women parishioners, to inspect the bodies and form an opinion. Whereas many of the common causes of death left stigmata that were plain for all to see, e.g. plague and smallpox, other diseases gave rise to less definite changes and there was doubtless considerable guesswork on the part of the searchers.

When the secular authorities made the registration of vital events mandatory, a government department called the Registrar General's Office was established to supervise the processing and collation of records, and to report to Parliament and other government departments. Dr William Farr was the first medical statistician at the office. His meticulous and imaginative analyses of the data set the standards for the present sophisticated system for the registration, analysis and publication of vital events. Now the task of collating, analysing and publishing information relating to vital events is the responsibility of the OPCS.

Births

All births must be registered by one of the parents (or someone on their behalf) with the local Registrar of Births, Marriages and Deaths within 6 weeks of the event. Certain of the information required at this time is entered in the register and is available for public scrutiny. This is:

child's name, sex, date and place of birth, and legitimacy;

mother's name, place of birth and usual residence;

father's name (if known), place of birth and occupation.

Not all of these data are entered on the birth certificate. Additional confidential information is collected for statistical purposes. This includes mother's date of birth and father's date of birth (if his name appears on the register). For legitimate births, the following additional information is required: date of parents' marriage, number of previous marriages of the mother and number of children born in the present marriage, distinguishing those born dead from those born alive.

If the child is *still born*, a certificate of cause of still birth has to be presented to the registrar. This certificate is similar to a death certificate and is issued either by a registered medical practitioner or by a state certified midwife involved with the birth.

Tabulations and analyses of birth data are published annually by OPCS. They are used to study patterns of fertility and to assist in making population estimates and projections.

Deaths

The present regulations governing registration of deaths were set out in the Births and Deaths Registration Act (1968). The Act requires that:

> . . . in the case of the death of any person who has been attended during his last illness by a registered medical practitioner, that practitioner shall sign a certificate . . . stating to the best of his knowledge and belief the cause of death and shall forthwith deliver that certificate to the Registrar.

The certificate that the doctor is required to complete and sign (Fig. 8.2) is one of cause of death, not of fact, since the doctor is not obliged to inspect the body after death. After giving the patient's name, age, date and place of death and details of how far the death was investigated, the doctor is required to state the 'immediate cause' of death. There is then space provided for him to record the 'antecedent causes' (giving the 'underlying cause' last) and any other significant conditions that may have contributed to the death. As far as possible the doctor should use generally accepted terminology, such as that set out in the International Classification of Disease (ICD). The Registrar requires him to avoid the use of indefinite and ambiguous terms such as 'heart failure' or 'old age'. The completion of the certificate is quite straightforward in the case of an individual who has died as a result of a well defined disease that has been extensively investigated in life, e.g. death by bronchopneumonia due to carcinomatosis due to carcinoma of the bronchus, with chronic bronchitis as a significant condition that contributed to death. However, in many circumstances the death certificate cannot be completed with precision, e.g. in the case of an old person who has previously had a stroke, has diabetes, has chronic cardiac failure, is known to have bronchitis, has been bedridden for months and who is found dead in bed one morning. In such cases the certified cause of death is an arbitrary opinion rather than a statement of fact. Generally the precision of death certification tends to diminish with increasing age of the deceased.

An informant, who is usually a close relative of the deceased, a person present at death, the person in charge of the institution in which the person died or the person responsible for the disposal of the body, must register the death with the Registrar as soon after death as possible. When doing so he or she must give the following information:

Side 1

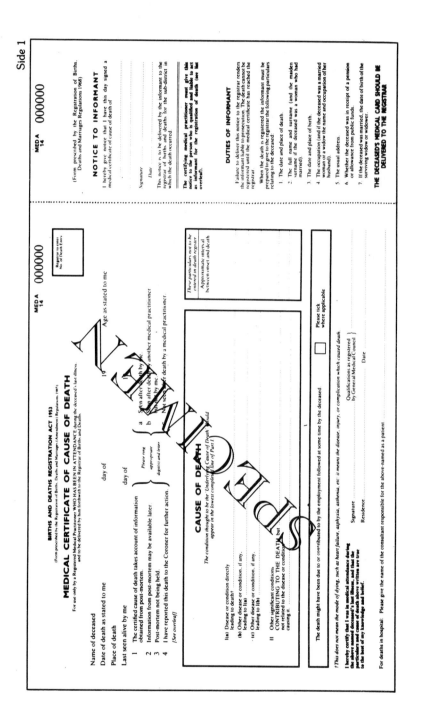

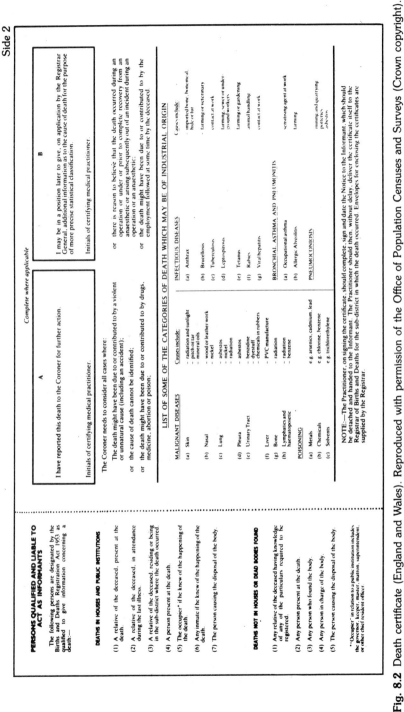

Fig. 8.2 Death certificate (England and Wales). Reproduced with permission of the Office of Population Censuses and Surveys (Crown copyright).

date and place of death;
full name and sex of deceased;
maiden name of married woman;
date and place of birth of deceased;
occupation and usual address of deceased.

These data are recorded in the register. If the Registrar is satisfied that the particulars are in order and that there is no need to report the death to the coroner he will issue a death certificate and authority for burial.

Death registration data are collated and analysed by the OPCS. The causes of death that are analysed are normally those given as the *underlying cause* rather than the *immediate cause* because the former is more informative and more useful for the study of disease in the community. In the first example given above, the death would be classified as due to carcinoma of the bronchus. The tables published by OPCS must be interpreted with this rule in mind. They do not necessarily provide a true picture of mortality attributable in whole or part to specific causes.

In certain circumstances a normal death certificate cannot be issued. These are when there was no medical attendant during the last illness of the deceased, when it is suspected that the death resulted from unnatural causes, or when the death occurred before full recovery from a surgical operation or the administration of an anaesthetic. In such circumstances it must be reported to the coroner either by the attending doctor, or the police or the Registrar. A *Coroner* is a member of the judiciary and is bound by legal processes. He has to be legally qualified but not necessarily medically qualified, though some have both qualifications. The Coroner investigates the death by enquiry, either directly or through his officers. He may order a post-mortem examination and he may hold an inquest, with or without a jury. Having established the cause of death he will then sign a death certificate. It should be noted that it is the Coroner's job to establish the cause of death, not who caused the death. If he has reason to believe that death was caused by the unlawful action of another person, he is bound to forward the papers to the Director of Public Prosecutions.

If those responsible for the disposal of the body wish the deceased to be cremated, an additional certificate is required. The person wishing to have the body cremated has to complete part of a form. The practitioner who attended the deceased during the last illness completes another part. This part has certain similarities to a certificate of cause of death but the doctor must have inspected the body after death. The third part is completed by another practitioner who is not professionally associated with the attending practitioner nor related to him or to the deceased. He must have been on the Medical Register for at least 5 years. This second doctor must inspect the body and form the view that the cause of death is as stated by the other practitioner. The final part is completed by the medical referee of crematoria for the local government authority involved. He has to affirm that the particulars on the other parts of the form are reasonable and have been completed by properly qualified doctors.

Abortions

Since the Abortion Act (1967) came into force it has been permissible for a pregnancy to be terminated provided it has not progressed beyond 28 weeks gestation *if* two doctors believe that the continuation of the pregnancy would be injurious to the physical or mental health of the woman or that there is a risk that the child may be born with a handicap that would prevent it from leading a normal life. Under 1990 legislation abortion is normally permissible only up to 24 weeks gestation. When a termination of pregnancy is carried out under the provision of the Act (it is illegal to terminate a pregnancy other than for reasons set out in the Act) the doctors involved have a statutory obligation to notify the Department of Health (DoH, formerly the DHSS). The form of notification asks for the name, date of birth and marital status of the woman, her normal place of residence, the number of previous pregnancies, distinguishing those that proceeded to term from those that were terminated. The presumed duration of the pregnancy, the statutory grounds for the operation and the place where it was carried out are also required. The forms are sent in confidence to the DoH where they are checked to ensure that the law is not being abused. They are collated and analysed by OPCS which publishes annual tabulations setting out the number of abortions by different criteria.

Morbidity

General

Morbidity statistics are concerned with the amount and types of illness that occur in the community. Most routinely collected morbidity data suffer from serious shortcomings partly because of the ephemeral nature and imprecise diagnosis of many illnesses and partly because of inadequacies in the information systems. Consequently although they should give a more complete picture of the incidence of disease in communities than mortality data, they do so with varying reliability and must be interpreted with caution.

One of the principal problems centres around the definition of illness itself. For some people, a common cold or backache may represent an 'illness' and justify them seeking medical help or being away from work. These people's illnesses may be recorded in one of the many routine data systems. For other people, symptoms that the medical profession would regard as indicative or diagnostic of major disease may be regarded as having no serious significance, an inconvenience to be tolerated until normal recovery takes place. Because they do not seek medical aid nor allow the symptoms to alter their lifestyle, e.g. take time off from work they will not feature in any morbidity statistics.

Another problem is that diagnostic precision varies between doctors according to their perception of the disease that they are treating. For example, influenza and upper respiratory viral infections in most people are minor, self-limiting conditions for which there is no specific treatment. Diagnostic precision is unnecessary and it is time-wasting to attempt to discriminate between the many causes by complicated and expensive viral studies and other examinations. In such circumstances the data that are generated may not have sufficient precision for epidemiological studies.

In many cases the stage at which disease is treated depends on a complex series of factors other than the patient's perception of the problem. These include the availability of health service treatments, e.g. waiting lists, out-patient appointment availability, etc and the acceptability of the treatments that the patient believes will be offered. This will affect the morbidity recorded at hospitals and employment sickness absence figures.

Finally, there is a quite separate problem in the way morbidity statistics are calculated and presented. The calculation of mortality rates is relatively straightforward because each individual can only die once. Thus, if there are 10 deaths in a population of 162, the death rate is 61.7 per thousand. If, however, ten episodes of an illness occur amongst 162 persons during a year it does not mean that 61.7 per thousand population were ill; one individual may have had more than one episode of illness; indeed, all the episodes may have occurred in the same individual. Many morbidity statistics are collected in such a way that it is impossible to distinguish episodes from individuals. When presenting or making use of rates it is important to be clear how the rate was derived.

Routine statistics

The principal morbidity statistics recorded routinely in England and Wales are:
- discharges from non-psychiatric (general) hospitals;
- admissions to psychiatric hospitals and hospitals for the mentally handicapped;
- statutory notifications of infectious diseases;
- notification of episodes of sexually transmitted diseases;
- notification of 'prescribed' and other industrial disease and accidents;
- notification of congenital malformations;
- registration of handicapped persons;
- cancer registration.

Hospital discharges (non-psychiatric)

In the late 1950s a system was established for the collection of detailed information on a random 10% sample of patients discharged (including deaths) from all NHS hospitals in England and Wales except those hospitals exclusively used for mental illness or mental handicap and convalescence units. The purpose of the system, the *Hospital In-Patient Enquiry (HIPE)*, was to measure morbidity and bed occupancy, to monitor trends in medical practice and to provide information essential for planning the health service. From the early 1970s many hospitals began to use a more sophisticated system for collecting these data, called *Hospital Activity Analysis (HAA)*. The principal difference between HAA and HIPE was that *all* discharges and deaths in hospitals were included. All the information recorded by HIPE was collected with some additional information.

The data collected were of two types. The first characterizes the patient (date of birth, sex, occupation, address, source of referral, etc). The second was concerned with the admission itself (the specialty, consultant, diagnoses, treatment, dates of admission and discharge and whether the patient died or not). There is a special form for maternity cases which, in addition to giving details of the delivery, gives details of the baby.

The HIPE data from all hospitals were collated and analysed by the OPCS and annual reports were published jointly by them and the DHSS (now the DoH). Serial data from these systems are available for 1968–1987.

Although both HIPE and HAA should have produced accurate data on the work of hospitals and provided useful indices of morbidity for many illnesses, neither system was entirely satisfactory. The quality of the information that was actually available was substantially dependent upon the enthusiasm of the staff and doctors who were responsible for the completion of the forms. There is evidence that forms were not submitted for the correct sample for HIPE or for all patients in the case of hospitals using HAA. Amongst the forms that were submitted some of the data did not agree with the information in the patients' clinical records. The problems did not usually arise from lack of care or diligence so much as from the fact that the systems were separate from patient care and hospital management. Moreover, the information generated tended to be too little and was produced too late to have any practical effect on the management of the hospital's resources. Nevertheless the data collected through these systems over many years provide useful indices of morbidity. They are now being displaced by data generated by semi-integrated district based information systems. These newer computer dependent systems are designed to produce comprehensive managerial and other information in line with the recommendations of the Korner Committee, a special committee set up by the DoH (see p. 81).

Psychiatric in-patient admissions (Mental Health Enquiry)

Mental hospital admissions present somewhat different problems from those of non-psychiatric hospitals because the length of stay may run into many years. If the data were collected on discharges, as in the general hospitals, then the information could be misleading about the current level of morbidity and working practices of psychiatrists. However, if only admission data were collected, then no information on activities during the admission would be available nor would the definitive diagnosis. Thus, since 1964, data on all psychiatric admissions and all discharges have been collected and analysed. The analysis and reporting on these data is undertaken by the DoH. Reports are published by the DoH at regular intervals. Statistics on mentally handicapped admissions are collected in a similar way.

The data suffer from the same shortcomings as HAA and HIPE data for similar reasons. The Mental Health Enquiry (MHE) is being replaced by the District Information System (see p. 81).

Infectious diseases

When a doctor suspects that a patient is suffering from a notifiable infectious disease or from food poisoning (Table 8.1) the law requires him to send a

Table 8.1 Notifiable diseases.

Under the Public Health (Control of Disease) Act 1984

Cholera	Smallpox
Plague	Typhus
Relapsing fever	

Under the Public Health (Infectious Diseases) Regulations 1988

Acute encephalitis	Ophthalmia neonatorum
Acute poliomyelitis	Paratyphoid fever
Anthrax	Rabies
Diphtheria	Rubella
Dysentery (amoebic or bacillary)	Scarlet fever
Leprosy	Tetanus
Leptospirosis	Tuberculosis
Malaria	Typhoid fever
Measles	Viral haemorrhagic fever
Meningitis	Viral hepatitis
Meningococcal septicaemia	Whooping cough
(without meningitis)	Yellow fever
Mumps	

Note AIDS is not a statutorily notifiable disease. Instead doctors are urged to participate in a voluntary confidential reporting scheme. Cases of AIDS should be reported on a special AIDS clinical report form in *strict medical confidence* to the Director of the PHLS CDSC.

certificate to the local medical officer responsible for infectious disease control immediately. The medical officer responsible for infectious disease control is usually the Medical Officer for Environmental Health (MOEH). When it is a disease that is likely to require urgent control measures to be taken, the doctor will normally notify the MOEH by telephone and provide the formal certificate later. Similar action will usually be taken in the case of non-notifiable infectious diseases (or outbreaks due to other causes, e.g. chemical poisoning) which may require immediate epidemiological investigation.

The importance of complete and prompt notification is not universally appreciated and therefore many infectious diseases are under-reported. Notification is important for a variety of purposes. In the case of some infections, such as food and waterborne disease (food poisoning/typhoid, etc), bacterial meningitis (particularly meningococcal infection), infectious hepatitis, diphtheria and Lassa and other viral haemorrhagic fevers immediate action may be required to limit the spread of infection and to safeguard the public health. Notifications are also of value in studying the aetiological factors influencing the incidence of disease in the community and in monitoring the efficacy of vaccination and immunization and other programmes.

Notifications of episodes of sexually transmitted diseases

Sexually transmitted disease (STD) clinics of the NHS in the UK are required to make regular returns to the DoH (or equivalent health department) of the numbers of new attendances. The cases are notified under the following headings:

syphilis;

gonorrhea;

non-specific genital infection;

trichomoniasis;

candidiasis;

scabies;

pediculosis pubis;

herpes simplex;

condylomata acuminata;

molluscum contagiosum;

chancroid;

lymphogranuloma venereum;

granuloma inguinale;

and all other *attendances* whether or not treatment was required. For two of these diseases, syphilis and gonorrhea, the age of the patient and whether the disease was contracted outside the country has to be stated. In no cases are any data that identify individuals given.

Although this system provides a useful picture of the overall trends in STD it has to be appreciated that not all cases treated are seen in NHS STD clinics. The nature of the information that is collected means that it is of limited value for all but the most basic of epidemiological studies. Notifications of HIV infection or AIDS are not included in STD clinic reports. Details of cases of AIDS are reported separately in confidence to the Director of the Communicable Disease Surveillance Centre in London, which also collates reports from laboratories on HIV antibody positive cases.

Industrial diseases and accidents

In order to improve personal safety at places of work, the Health and Safety Executive (HSE) was established as a statutory body in 1974. Doctors are required to inform the CEHO of the local civil authority of the occurrence of any of the notifiable diseases they list. Doctors must also report poisoning by the following substances:

aniline

arsenic

benzene (chronic)

berylium

cadmium

carbon bisulphide

compressed air

chrome

lead

manganese

mercury

phosphorous

Also cases of epitheliomatosis, toxic anaemia and toxic jaundice.

The HSE publishes the reported figures annually. Although the system is of great value in controlling these diseases, it undoubtedly gives an underestimate of the true incidence of these conditions. Many of the diseases occur in factories and work places in which there is no medical officer and even when detected by another doctor, cases that occur in such places are not always reported.

Employers also have an obligation to notify the HSE of accidents (both fatal and non-fatal) which occur in their factories or work place. These are published in the annual report.

A third source of data relating to industrial diseases is notifications of *prescribed occupational diseases*, e.g. pneumoconiosis in coal miners, tuberculosis in medical laboratory workers and mesothelioma in asbestos workers. Workers who have these diseases are entitled to compensation under current regulations. This notification is thus probably more complete than that for many other diseases since there is a potential advantage in doing so to the individual with the disease. There are currently about 50 prescribed occupational diseases.

Congenital malformations

A national scheme for the notification of congenital malformations was instituted in England and Wales in 1961 after the thalidomide episode. Although there is no statutory requirement on doctors or midwives to notify cases, the scheme seems to work well and has produced useful data. One of the problems with these data is the definition of malformations. There is little difficulty in detecting a major malformation but some minor abnormalities may not be noticed, or if noticed are not deemed to be of sufficient importance to justify notification.

Handicapped persons

Local authorities, through their social service departments, are required to maintain registers of persons covered by the Chronic Sick and Disabled Persons Act (1970). Disabilities include the blind and partially sighted, the deaf, the mentally handicapped and those with a disability of locomotion.

Cancer registration

Malignant disease has long been a major cause of morbidity and mortality in this and in most other countries. In order to study these diseases it is essential to know the numbers of people affected by different forms of cancer and their survival rates. The system of cancer registration was set up specifically to facilitate research in this field. Each region of the NHS maintains a *cancer register* to which new cases are notified by hospitals and others. The OPCS also notifies each Regional Cancer Registry of all persons who die from malignant disease in their region. Data from all regions are analysed further by OPCS. Periodic official reports are published giving detailed tabulations of incidence, survival and mortality rates for various malignant diseases at different stages.

Other sources of data

Hospital out-patients

Until full implementation of the new District Information Systems (DIS) (see p. 81) the only regularly recorded out-patient data are the numbers of old and new patients attending by clinic specialty. There is some inconsistency between hospitals in the designation of clinics, e.g. in some hospitals 'neurology' may be combined with 'general medicine'; 'rheumatology' is often interchangeable with 'physical medicine'. Summaries of data on hospital out-patient activity are published in the *Digest of Health and Personal Social Service Statistics.*

General practice

There have been several national morbidity surveys in general practice since the health service began; each carried out in the years around national censuses. Selected general practitioners recorded consultations, episodes of illness and diagnoses, and the age and sex of the patients consulting in their practice during a 1 year period. The practices which took part in these enquires all volunteered and therefore the results may not be applicable to the whole population. Nevertheless they provide valuable information about morbidity and patterns of use of health services.

Prescriptions issued by general practitioners

NHS prescription forms are forwarded by the dispenser each month to the Central Pricing Bureau. After pricing, a one-in-two-hundred sample is analysed by ingredient and by cost within each standard region of the country. The analysis of prescription data is primarily for administrative and accounting purposes. It can also be used for certain types of morbidity investigation.

Laboratory reports

The Communicable Disease Surveillance Centre (CDSC) of the Public Health Laboratory Service (PHLS) receives weekly reports from microbiology laboratories in England and Wales on cases of laboratory diagnosed infections. The amount of clinical and epidemiological data reported varies depending on the infection. Although the data are incomplete and lack denominators which prevents their use to calculate incidence rates, they provide a useful means of monitoring trends and detecting outbreaks. The CDSC also collects data related to infectious disease from other sources, e.g. reports of outbreak investigations and immunization statistics. These reports are collated and published in the *Weekly Communicable Disease Report.*

General Household Survey (GHS)

This is an on-going survey of a random sample of private households in England and Wales designed to provide some detailed social statistics. Many of the questions included in the survey relate to illness, disability and the utilization of health services. Reports of the GHS are published annually by the OPCS.

INDICES OF HEALTH AND DISEASE

The health of the community can be measured by the appropriate use of the basic data from sources described in the previous section. To be intelligible, however, the crude numbers need to be presented in a form that allows valid comparisons to be made between groups, between years and between different areas. There are certain conventions in the handling and presentation of data.

Types of variable

There are three main types of variable:

qualitative;

continuous quantitative;

discrete quantitative.

Qualitative variables

These are descriptive of a fixed attribute. Examples are sex, religion, occupation and nationality. Such data are sometimes classified for convenience by using numbers, e.g. 1 = male, 2 = female: 1 = Church of England, 2 = Roman Catholic, 3 = Methodist, etc. These numbers have no meaning other than as a label.

Continuous quantitative variables

These measure attributes that can occur at any point on a scale, e.g. height and weight. The degree of precision to which a continuous variable is measured, depends upon its intended use in a particular investigation and the discriminatory power of the measuring instrument.

Discrete quantitative variables

These measure attributes that can occur only as whole numbers (integers), e.g. the number of children born to a woman or the number of deaths in a year.

Grouping of data

For convenience of handling and presentation, continuous variables may be grouped as if they were discrete, e.g. height to the nearest centimetre, group all those whose height is over 122.5 cm and under 123.5 cm, all over 123.5 cm and under 124.5 cm, etc. Discrete variables may also be grouped to produce larger numbers in each category. The class intervals between successive groups should usually be equal but it is often convenient to group all values at the extreme end of a scale.

Situations in which groupings are natural should be distinguished from those where they are arbitrary, e.g. 'under 16 years' and '16 years and over' could be regarded as natural grouping in as much as people in the former category cannot be married and those in the latter can. For other variables, e.g. blood pressure, there is no such natural division. It is possible arbitrarily to define blood pressure in excess of 130 mmHg as high and below that level as not high, but this does not necessarily have any significance. Quantitative data rarely fall into natural categories.

Rates

It is rarely useful to state numbers of events observed and recorded alone. These can be interpreted only when they are related to a denominator, i.e. expressed as a rate, e.g. it is not helpful to say that the number of deaths from pneumoconiosis is greater in coal miners than in, say, farm workers without relating the figures to the numbers of people employed in the two occupations, nor that one type of operation is followed by more cases of sepsis than another without knowing how many of each is performed.

Two types of rate are frequently used:

Events related to the population, or sub-group of it, in which they occur

Examples

A birth rate is usually given as x per thousand total population per year. Age-specific rates relate the number of events in persons in a specified age group to the total population in that age group, e.g. y deaths per thousand men aged 45–64 years per year. Cause-specific rates relate cases of a specified disease to the population at risk, e.g. z cases of stroke per thousand hypertensive patients per year. Such rates must *always* have a specified time dimension.

Special events related to total events

Examples

Still births are usually expressed as x per thousand total births. Operative mortality can be expressed as y deaths per thousand operations. Case fatality rates relate the number of deaths from a particular illness to the total number of cases of that illness. This type of rate is *not* time dimensioned because the time dimension is always the same for the numerator as it is for the denominator. ·

Incidence and prevalence rates

In order to demonstrate how incidence and prevalence rates are derived, the mortality and morbidity experience of the employees in a hypothetical factory is shown schematically in Fig. 8.3.

Incidence rates

The *incidence* of a disease or other events is the number of new cases that occur during a specified period in a defined population. Thus, from Fig. 8.3 in year B, the incidence of illness was 8. (The first illness in subject 11 and the illnesses in subjects 14, 19 and 20 started before the beginning of the period specified and are therefore discounted.) The incidence rate is 8 per 18 persons per year (by convention the mid-year population is used as the denominator). It should be noted that the incidence for a specific period is only valid for that period. Thus in the 6 months January – June of year B, the incidence of disease was 5; it is clear that it cannot be multiplied to give an incidence of 10 during a 12-month period.

Prevalence rates

The *prevalence* of a disease is the number of cases in the population at a particular point in time, *point prevalence*, or during a specified period, *period prevalence*. Both are expressed as a rate (x per thousand population). From Fig. 8.3 the point prevalence rate at the beginning of the year was 4 per 17 persons and at the beginning of August it was 2 per 16 persons (three had died since the beginning of the year and two had joined). The period prevalence for the year was 12 per 18 persons (by convention the denominator is the mid-year population). The period prevalence approximates to the sum of the point prevalence at the beginning of the period and the incidence during the period.

Standardization of rates

Rates calculated by using the total number of events as the numerator and the total population as the denominator are called *crude rates*. Their value is limited, particularly when comparing two populations with different age structures. In these circumstances it is essential to adjust the data to take account of the differences, this is called *age standardization*. The two methods of standardization most frequently used are *indirect* standardization and *direct* standardization.

Indirect standardization

The conventional method of indirect standardization for age is to calculate the *standardized mortality ratio (SMR)*. The SMR compares the mortality (either from a specific disease or for all causes) which occurred in a designated group

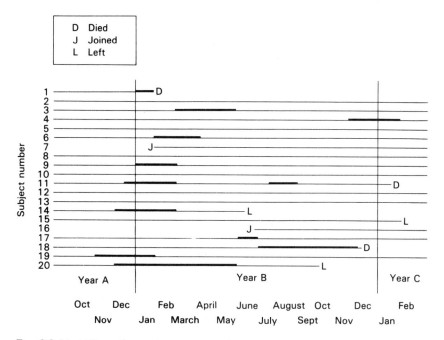

Fig. 8.3 Morbidity and mortality experienced in a hypothetical factory.

with that of a standard population. It is the ratio (usually expressed as a percentage) of the number of deaths which occurred in the designated group to the number that would have been expected if the mortality rates in each age band of the designated group had been the same as those of the standard population.

The death rates for each age and sex group in the standard population (M_x) are multiplied by the number of persons of that age and sex in the population being investigated (P_x). This gives the 'expected' number of deaths in that particular age/sex group. The expected deaths for each age/sex group are then added to give the 'expected' number of deaths in the whole population being investigated. The observed number of deaths (D) is then divided by the expected deaths to give the SMR:

$$SMR = \frac{\text{Observed deaths } [D]}{\text{Expected deaths } [\Sigma(P_x \times M_x)]} \times 100$$

Examples

Members of the armed forces tend to be younger than the male population of the country as a whole. Therefore the fact that they tend to have a lower mortality is not illuminating. It is of interest to examine the mortality of this occupational group after taking account of the age factor. Their SMR for ischaemic heart disease is calculated in Table 8.2.

This indicates that mortality from ischaemic heart disease amongst men in the armed forces after adjusting for age distribution is higher than the male population as a whole by a factor of 1.73.

Table 8.2 Mortality from ischaemic heart disease in men serving in the armed forces.

Age group (years)	Death rates from ischaemic heart disease in England and Wales (per 1000) (M_x)	Population of armed services (1000s) (P_x)	Expected deaths $(M_x \times P_x)$	Observed deaths
15–24	0	165.03	0	1
25–34	0.06	73.24	4.39	6
35–44	0.50	42.25	21.13	22
45–54	2.01	15.93	32.02	43
55–64	6.05	4.67	28.75	76
Total			85.79	148

$$SMR = \frac{\text{Observed}}{\text{Expected}} \times 100 = \frac{148 \times 100}{85.79} = 173$$

This indicates that mortality from ischaemic heart disease amongst forces personnel is higher than the national experience.

Note SMRs for occupational sub-groups are usually confined to persons aged 15–64 years because the working population is confined to this age group.

Another example of how standardization can be helpful is in comparing mortality in different years. The age structure of England and Wales has been changing for many years and therefore crude death rates can give a misleading impression of changes in mortality. The SMR gives a clearer indication of the true picture (Table 8.3).

Table 8.3 Mortality in males in England and Wales in 1965 compared with 1973.

Age group (years)	Death rate (per 1000) males in England and Wales, 1965 (M_x)	Male population in England and Wales (1000s) 1973 (P_x)	Expected deaths $(P_x \times M_x)$	Observed deaths
<1	21.8	355.3	7746.0	
1–4	0.9	1561.7	1406.0	
5–14	0.5	4037.3	2019.0	
15–24	1.0	3534.2	3534.0	
25–34	1.1	3337.5	3671.0	
35–44	2.5	2877.6	7194.0	
45–54	7.4	3033.6	22449.0	
55–64	21.4	2643.1	56562.0	
65–74	53.0	1855.9	98363.0	
75 +	118.4	639.7	75740.0	
85 +	242.4	112.8	27343.0	
Total			306026.0	296546

$$SMR = \frac{Observed}{Expected} \times 100 = \frac{296546}{306026} = 97$$

This indicates that mortality in males in England and Wales declined between 1965 and 1973.

Direct standardization

Direct standardization for age involves calculating the age-specific death rates in the study population and applying them to a 'standard' population, this can be real or hypothetical. In this way the number of deaths that would have occurred in the standard population had it experienced the same death rates as the study population, can be computed and compared with other groups. The method of direct standardization is shown in Table 8.4.

Error in health information

The value of data ultimately depends on how accurately they reflect the true frequency of the disease (or other variable being measured) in the population concerned. This section sets out some of the common sources of error that may affect routine health information and the steps which can be taken to reduce their effects.

Errors affecting mortality and morbidity rates are of two kinds:
those affecting the numerator;
those affecting the denominator.

Table 8.4 Standardization of mortality in England and Wales in 1949 against the 1979 population.

Age group	Population 1949 (a) (1000s)	Deaths 1949 (b)	Death rate (1949) (b/a)	1979 Population (c) (1000s)	Expected deaths (c × b/a)
0–9	3417	17643	5.16	3339	17231.3
10–19	2869	2345	0.82	4063	3331.7
20–29	3339	5031	1.51	3534	5336.3
30–39	3189	6839	2.14	3326	7117.6
40–49	3178	16062	5.05	2020	14241.0
50–59	2335	32097	13.75	2924	40205.0
60–69	1727	60580	35.08	2257	74661.6
70–79	957	77127	80.59	1384	111536.6
80 +	228	42218	185.17	355	65735.4
Total	21239	260278		24002	339396.5

The age-standardized 1949 death rate (against the 1979 population) is 339396.5/24002 = 14.14 per thousand. This can be compared directly with the crude death rate for 1979 (12.41).

Numerator error

The number of recorded cases of a particular disease may be in error for many reasons including the following.

• *Diagnostic inaccuracy*

This is affected by the training, skills and interests of the attending physician, advances in medical knowledge of pathogenesis, variations in the criteria accepted in defining a diagnosis, differences in the availability and use of special investigations.

• *Incomplete identification of cases*

The probability that patients will consult a doctor is influenced by such factors as past medical history, cultural and social background, occupation, economic constraints, e.g. paid sick leave, availability of medical care — which is related to numbers of doctors, distance from doctor's surgery, number of hospital beds and appointments systems. (The effect of variations in illness behaviour is most marked in mild, non-fatal and self-limiting conditions.)

• *The recording system*

The completeness and comparability of different sources of data may be affected by the doctor's view of the value of records, the simplicity and efficiency of a records system, changes in the conventions for coding and classification of disease or rules for selecting priorities among multiple diagnoses.

Denominator error

The size of population at risk often cannot be accurately defined and various methods of estimation have to be used. Some reasons for this are:

• *population migration* between censuses may increase or decrease the size of population within an area;

- *changes in population structure* within different areas, e.g. age, race, occupational distribution, due to migration, changing fertility patterns, housing and industrial decay or development;
- *changes in administrative boundaries* for reasons that may or may not relate to health and the provision of health services.

Reduction of error in routine statistics

The effects of errors such as those above can be reduced by:
- use of a standard diagnostic classification such as the ICD when recording mortality or modifications of this for morbidity;
- combination of diagnostic categories between which transposition of cases may occur, e.g. cancer of the colon and large bowel obstruction;
- use of standard recording and registration procedures;
- use of denominator populations derived from similar sources and compiled by comparable procedures.

Errors in routine statistics can rarely be completely eliminated. Therefore caution is needed in their interpretation, particularly between different localities and at different times (see also Chapter 4).

Health information systems

Information systems are used to assemble facts and figures from a variety of sources for analysis. Their main purposes are to provide accurate knowledge of the incidence and prevalence of disease in a community which will assist in the organization and monitoring of its health services and in disease surveillance activities. Ideally every health event and every kind of health resource would be recorded in a systematic and instantly available form. In practice this is neither possible nor desirable as it would require an enormously complex and expensive system which would be too slow and cumbersome to be of value. Most health information systems have been developed to meet particular needs. Nevertheless, unfortunately the data are often inaccurate and the system does not always allow user's questions to be answered with ease. These shortcomings tend to bring systems into disrepute and the enthusiasm for collecting data (as well as making use of it) wanes.

Problems of information systems

Some of the commonly encountered problems of information systems are as follows.

Lack of motivation among recorders

Often a low priority is accorded to the task of record keeping. This leads to delays in completion and poor quality of records, e.g. inaccurate information, items missing or no record at all. For these reasons all arrangements for 'data capture', as it is called, should be simple to operate and create the minimum amount of work.

Design of data capture procedure

The type of record needed for an information system is not always compatible with that required for clinical purposes. It is, however, often possible to use records made for other purposes if they are carefully designed, i.e. standard format, provision for coding, etc. This requires a degree of collaboration between different interests which it is often hard to achieve.

Inflexibility in the system

The need for simplicity in records means that the number of items recorded has to be restricted. Some flexibility can be gained by allowing room on the record for additional items of local interest beyond a set of basic data required of all recorders.

Irrelevance of analyses

Users may feel that standard analyses tell them nothing new or are unhelpful in solving their problems. This tends to sap enthusiasm for the system.

In the design of a routine information system, therefore, the following requirements should be met:

- the intended uses of the system should be specified so that the data recorded will be appropriate to their purpose and the collection of irrelevant data can be avoided;
- the recording procedures should be standardized and the data collected should be easy to obtain, accurate and as complete as possible in order that reliable comparisons can be made over periods of time and between different places;
- data should be collected from all relevant sources for collation and analysis at a central point;
- there should be well organized provision for data storage, updating, processing and retrieval;
- the system should be capable of providing answers to enquiries within the field for which it is designed with speed and accuracy.

District Information Systems (DIS)

By the late 1970s it was clear that the then current major information systems used by the NHS (HAA, HIPE and the MHE) were able to provide neither the optimum data nor data of good enough quality to meet the planning and management requirements of the service. Moreover the rapid developments in information technology made it possible to be more ambitious in the design and implementation of information systems than had been possible 20 years previously. In 1980 the Secretary of State for Health and Social Services appointed a working party to review the existing health service information systems and recommend changes and developments. The working party was known as the Korner Committee (after the name of its chairman). The Korner Committee published a series of reports and most of its recommendations are being implemented.

The principle developed by the Committee is that health districts should have computer-based integrated patient-based information systems covering all aspects of health service activity, namely:

hospital in-patients and out-patients;

laboratory and scientific services;

paramedical services;

community health services;

health service manpower;

management accounting;

In order to encourage the collection of high quality data, the systems that are being implemented are designed to produce the management (and epidemiological) data automatically as the normal patient management, laboratory and scientific tasks are being performed. In the past the collection of data had been a separate exercise that had little relevance to the day to day work of the hospital or community services. In pursuance of this policy sophisticated computer technology is being introduced into all departments in the hospitals and in many areas of medical practice in the community. At the same time most health districts are introducing a common patient numbering system in order to promote linkage of all records relating to the same patient whilst preserving confidentiality.

In their reports, the Korner Committee stressed the need to define a minimum data set for each area of activity and encouraged individual units to give careful consideration to what additional data would be of local value. They also stressed the need for more attention to be given to the analysis and presentation of data than there had been in the past.

It will be some years before integrated DISs are fully operational throughout the country. Once installed they will provide more sophisticated management information and much improved data for certain types of epidemiological study..

Surveillance

Disease surveillance is:
- the systematic and continuous collection of current data on the frequency of specific diseases and events that may influence their occurrence;
- the collation, analysis and interpretation of these data;
- the regular dissemination of the information to those responsible for disease control and service planning.

The purposes of a surveillance system are:
- to facilitate the early recognition of changes in the patterns of disease;
- to identify changes in environmental and host factors that may lead to an increase in the frequency of disease;
- to monitor the safety and effectiveness of preventive and control measures.

Computers in medicine

The advantages of computers over traditional methods of data processing are:
- the volume of data that can be handled economically is greater;

- the speed with which sophisticated processing can be undertaken is greatly increased.

Some of the present and possible future uses of computers in medicine include the following.

Individual patient care

- *On-line clinical record store.* All information on each patient is centrally recorded on a computer file. Since rapid and reliable access is essential, remote terminals for direct input and recall are required.
- *Patient management.* Treatment schedules, e.g. for radio-therapy, can be calculated and vital functions can be monitored, e.g. in intensive care units.
- *Laboratory investigations.* Readings from autoanalysers can be fed to the computer and individual results, e.g. in haematology, biochemistry, respiratory function, are calculated and printed out with predicted values in relation to patients' age, weight, height, etc.

Surveillance

Routine data are stored, analysed and tabulated. Indices are monitored for adverse trends, particularly increased incidence of disease above the epidemic threshold, e.g. cancer and congenital malformation registers, drug reactions, influenza morbidity and mortality.

Health service administration

The domestic management of a hospital can be improved, e.g. bed allocation, staff duty rotas, accounts and pay roll, inventories. Patient services can be organized and timetabled, e.g. out-patient appointments, scheduling of infant immunization, invitations to screening clinics of 'at risk' groups.

Research

Epidemiological research

- Routine statistical analysis and survey data tabulation;
- Building epidemic models and simulating alternative intervention strategies in order to predict their consequences
- Searching data for statistically significant correlations (caution is required in the interpretation of any particular level of significance in relation to the number of correlations tested).

Health care provision research

- Prediction of trends in need for services and their resources implications
- Devising organizational models
- Assessing alternative strategies in health care provision by simulation trials.

Record linkage

A serious disadvantage of most health information is that it is compiled from records of events as if they were isolated and discrete. There is no way to tell how many people are concerned or how any particular event relates to the subsequent history of the same person, especially if, for example, the patient is treated in more than one hospital. Records from various sources about medical and vital events for the same person are often brought together on an *ad hoc* basis for research purposes, e.g. in studies of survival rates in cancer patients. Computers now make it feasible for such record linkage to be carried out routinely on a large scale.

The principle of record linkage is that data on all specified events in a defined population are supplied to a central computer register where, by means of a unique identification number, each individual's personal record is regularly up-dated. The types of event commonly recorded are birth, marriage, death, hospital admission and discharge. Other useful data might include out-patient attendances, consultations with general practitioners, sickness absence from work, use of social services, prophylactic procedures and screening clinic attendances. The geographical areas covered and the population included on a register should be as wide as possible in order to reduce the risk of failing to record all the events or services received by each individual in a variety of locations.

Problems of record linkage

Size of data bank

The main problem is the volume of data that can accumulate and there is a limit to what can be stored, even on a computer file. Even if all the data could be stored, access to individual files and processing would become impossibly complex. Therefore, in practice, record linkage has been applied only on a limited scale.

Personal identification

Each individual requires a unique identification which is simple and reliable and consistently used.

Economics

The cost of maintaining a record linkage system on a national scale may not be justified in relation to the possible benefits.

Ethical and political

The recording of personal information on computer files is beset with ethical and political problems. Concern at the possible misuse of the data requires stringent safeguards to maintain confidentiality.

Uses of record linkage

Morbidity

Morbidity rates for persons can be calculated as well as for events. For example, the number of different people admitted to hospital can be identified as well as episodes of admission. Without linkage it is possible only to count admissions.

Prognosis

The course of events in individuals can be studied and this allows survival rates, recurrence rates and re-admission rates to be calculated. This is invaluable in evaluating treatment. Record linkage is also of value in tracing the histories of persons exposed to particular hazards, e.g. industrial processes, which are suspected of causing a specific disease.

Family and genetic studies

Record linkage facilitates the study of the frequency of particular conditions in members of the same family. In time it could show genetic inheritance patterns more clearly. It can also be used to show the relation between pre-natal events or disease and social factors in the mother (and father) and the subsequent health of the child.

Chapter 9
Medical Demography

Introduction

Despite the presence of many serious endemic diseases, the occurrence of major epidemics and wars, the populations of most European countries increased substantially during the past three to four hundred years. There has been a reduction in the rate of increase in recent decades and today the populations of most European and North American countries are relatively stable. It seems likely in the foreseeable future they will either remain stable or that there might even be a modest decrease.

The growth of the European resident population since the seventeenth century underestimates both the extent to which the numbers of European people increased and the rate at which the increase took place. Throughout the past four hundred years people have emigrated in large numbers mainly to the Americas, Australasia and to parts of Africa. The migrations were prompted by economic hardship, social pressures and religious persecution as well as for trading reasons and fortune hunting. The majority of the present populations of North America and Australasia are descendants of these migrants. Their numbers now exceed those of the parent (European) populations.

Whether or not the European population would have increased in size to the extent that it has without migration and dispersal throughout the world can only be a matter of speculation. It is unlikely that it would have done, as the natural resources of Europe would have been insufficient to support so large a population. Furthermore, the technology to create a safe urban environment, with pure water, adequate sanitation and means for the bulk transport of food, did not exist until recently.

The populations of most other parts of the world began to increase much more recently and their rate of increase has reached that prevailing in Europe in the eighteenth and nineteenth century only during the past few decades. An important difference between the contemporary situation in many of the poorer developing countries of the world and Europe in previous centuries is that there are no longer large, sparsely populated continents rich in natural resources that can be colonized and in which people can thrive. Thus, population growth, which in previous generations was regarded as a national problem, is now a world problem. It is widely believed that if the prevailing rates of growth are sustained, then the world's population, now about 4.5 thousand million, will double within the next 60 years. The earth's mineral and energy resources are finite and the rate at which they are being consumed is increasing, particularly by the industrialized countries. In many parts of the world there is a hopeless inability to meet local needs and resources are inadequate to enable them to import essential commodities. It is predicted that unless there is reduction in both the rate of population growth and the rate at which natural resources are consumed there will be a catastrophic failure to meet the basic needs of the majority of mankind within the next few generations.

Cataclysmic prophecies that mankind's future is threatened in this way are not new. They have been widely debated since the eighteenth century. Probably the best known writer associated with the problems of over-population is the Reverend Thomas Malthus, an eighteenth century English clergyman who attracted attention by his essay on 'The principles of population as it affects the future improvement of society'. The two principles from which he argued were: 'that food is necessary for the existence of man' and that 'the passion between the sexes is necessary and will remain nearly in its present state'. He argued that the power of the population to reproduce was greater than power of the earth to produce food. He concluded that there must be a 'strong and constantly operating check on population from the difficulty of subsistence'. This conclusion led him to recommend that there should be no extension of relief for the poor, as this would artificially reduce the difficulties of subsistence and lead to uncontrolled population growth. The time scale within which he predicted catastrophe was wrong, partly because he did not foresee emigration and colonization. His contention that difficulties in subsistence would act as a constant check on population growth has also been proved sadly wrong by the experience in the countries of Latin America, the Indian subcontinent and elsewhere.

At about the same time as the ideas of Malthus were being debated in Europe, similar discussions were taking place in China. Hung Wang Chi noted in 1793 that 'during a long reign of peace the government cannot prevent people from multiplying themselves, yet its remedies are few'. One of the solutions that he suggested was to legalize and encourage female infanticide, a practice that continues in some parts of the world to this day. Discussions of the problems of population have continued throughout the world up to the present time but now more is known about the size of the world population, the dynamics of growth and the potential resources of the earth. The United Nations, through its various agencies, now regards population growth as one of the major world problems that will affect the quality of life, health and survival of mankind.

The countries with high population growth are mainly the developing countries of the Third World where there are already regular famines, chronic poverty, frequent epidemics of crippling diseases and declining living standards. The situation will only be remedied if those countries with the highest growth rates in population achieve stability and the countries with the highest growth rates in consumption of resources reduce their demands.

The global problem of population growth is compounded by the fact that people are not evenly distributed on the habitable surface of the earth. Food shortages and disease are problems in some areas simply because of the local density of population rather than because the area as a whole has insufficient natural resources. It is important to recognize that health depends as much upon the systems for the distribution of food and water and the disposal of waste as it does upon the quantity of food produced or the availability of medical services.

Populations and growth rates

The size of the world's population and its growth rate is arrived at by collating data from every country. The quality of the data varies considerably from country to country. Most of the richer industrialized countries undertake regular and detailed censuses similar to those undertaken in England and Wales (see p. 60). They also have sophisticated and comprehensive systems for the registration of births, deaths and marriages. From these sources it is possible to build up a complete picture of the way in which the size and structure of the population changes.

In the poorer countries of the world national censuses are conducted infrequently and tend to be incomplete. The additional data that are required for demographic studies, the registration of vital events, are often defective. There are particular difficulties in the most deprived sections of these countries and amongst nomadic peoples or those living in sparsely populated regions of the world with poor communications. In these latter situations much of the data are available only on an irregular sample basis. It is not surprising that most of the work on population growth has used European data, because only in recent times has it been possible to study many of the other countries of the world.

The trends in population growth in England and Wales are not dissimilar to those in most European countries and can be used to illustrate the size and speed at which changes occurred. It has proved possible to estimate the number of residents at various times between 1100 and the early nineteenth century from analysis of ecclesiastical and governmental records. From the nineteenth century onwards census figures are available. The trend has been for the population to increase exponentially (Fig. 9.1). The temporary decreases in population due to major national disasters such as epidemics of plague are not discernible within

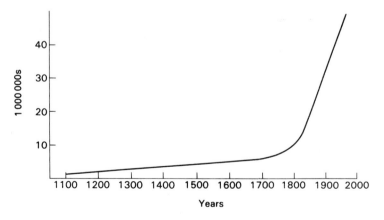

Fig. 9.1 The growth of population in England and Wales.

the scale used on this figure but at the time they had major impacts in some parts of the country. For example, Fig. 8.1, facing p. 60, shows the 'General Bills of Mortality for London' for 1641 and 1665. In both years the number of deaths greatly exceeded the number of births, in 1665 by a factor of 10. It should be remembered that Fig. 9.1 is solely concerned with the resident population and that during much of the period there was substantial migration. It should also be noted that the scale of the figure is such that the recent reduction in population growth rate is not apparent.

At the same time as the population increased its age structure changed. Figure 9.2 compares the age distribution of the population in 1821 with that in 1981. In 1821 the proportion of children was much greater than at the present time and the proportion of people over the age of 50 was considerably less. The 1981 census showed that the proportion of the population between 10 and 19 years is greater than that in the age group 0–9 years. This is due in part to an increase in the number of births during the 1960s and in part to a reduction in birth rates in the 1970s.

Clearly population can only increase if the number of births exceeds the number of deaths. The growth rate of human populations tends to be exponential because with each annual increase the proportion of the population potentially capable of reproduction increases. For this reason, the statement that there is an annual growth rate of x per thousand population (x being the difference between the birth rate and the death rate) gives a misleading impression of the magnitude of change. The conventional way of expressing growth is the population doubling time. This is the *theoretical* period that it will take for a given population to double, based upon the most recently available

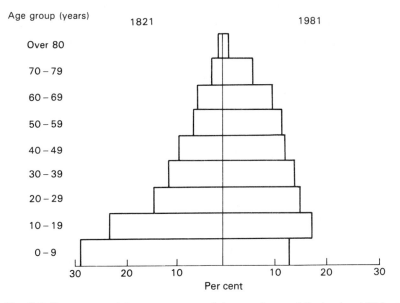

Fig. 9.2 Comparison of the age structure of the population of England and Wales in 1821 with that in 1981.

data. Clearly the doubling time will have to be revised when there is a change in either birth or death rates. The doubling time for the population of England and Wales, together with that for a number of other countries, is given in Table 9.1.

Table 9.1 Population doubling times.

Country	Population (in millions)	Growth rate per 1000 population	Population doubling time (years)
Brazil (1973)	101.71	28.3	25
India (1972)	563.49	26.1	27
Jamaica (1973)	1.87	24.1	29
USSR (1972)	249.75	9.0	77
USA (1973)	203.21	5.6	124
England and Wales (1973)	49.04	1.9	365

Demographic transition

The model of demographic transition provides a useful framework within which to consider the factors which determine changes in the size and structure of human populations. The population is stable both in size and in age structure when the birth and death rates are equal and static, irrespective of whether they are both high or both low. This phase is represented in Fig. 9.3 as period A. Typically primitive rural societies and poorly developed urban societies tend to have high birth and death rates. The highest mortality tends to be in infancy and childhood due to the combined effects of disease and poor nutrition.

Social progress and the introduction of industrial technology bring tangible and immediate benefits to the community. The most obvious are improvements in sanitation, in water supply and in the ability to distribute and store food. The immediate effect of these changes is that the chances of survival amongst the most vulnerable within the community, infants and children, are improved. Therefore the death rate begins to fall and the community enters phase B in Fig. 9.3. During this phase the crude birth rate actually rises because the proportion of the population that is capable of reproduction increases and there is little change in the age-specific birth rates. This is because people's reproduction behaviour tends to be learned from their parents and it can take several generations to adapt fully to new circumstances. In many societies the desirability of large families, which is a biological necessity for survival in pre-transitional communities, is formalized within the belief system of the group. For example, in many societies the number of children a man has is perceived as a measure of his virility.

The next phase (C in Fig. 9.3) is characterized by a decrease in the birth rate while the death rate continues to fall. Birth rates still exceed death rates and the exponential growth of the population, established in phase B, continues. Again this is because, despite a decrease in the average number of children born to each woman, there are more women in the reproductive age group than there were in the previous phase.

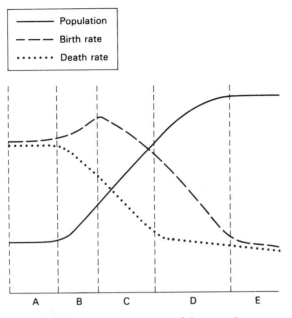

Fig. 9.3 Schematic representation of demographic transition.

Eventually death rates stabilize (phase D) but birth rates continue to fall. The transition of the society is completed in phase E, when birth and death rates are static and equal. By this time the size of the population is many times greater than it was in the pre-transitional phase. The size of the new stable population is determined by the speed of the transition.

Data from England and Wales can be used to illustrate the demographic changes discussed above. The crude and the age-specific death rates for selected age groups relative to the 1841 rates in England and Wales are shown in Fig. 9.4. The crude death rate is now about half what it was in the early nineteenth century. The greatest changes in mortality have been amongst the young, exemplified by the 5–9-year-olds in the figure, which are now less than 5% of the rates prevailing in the early nineteenth century. The smallest changes have been amongst the elderly. This is reflected in the change in life expectancy, another way of summarizing mortality, at different ages (Fig. 9.5). It is arrived at by applying the prevailing age and sex specific mortality rates to those people surviving to a particular age. It is clear that the greatest changes in life expectancy have been amongst the very young. Increased survival in the pre-reproductive age groups means that the proportion of the population capable of reproduction increases. Thus, although each age group of women may maintain the same age-specific fertility rates as previous generations, the crude birth rates will rise.

Reasons for the decline in mortality

The reduction in mortality in England and Wales since the nineteenth century is almost entirely due to the elimination of the major endemic infectious diseases

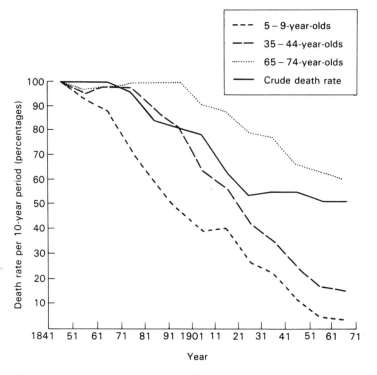

Fig. 9.4 Age-specific death rates per 10-year period for England and Wales since 1841, as percentage of the 1841–1850 age-specific rates.

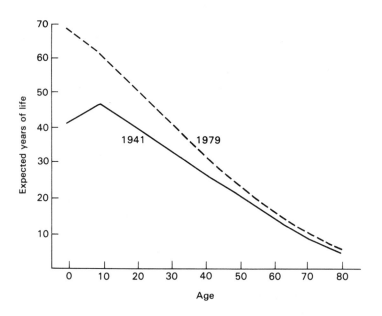

Fig. 9.5 Expectation of life at different ages in England and Wales in 1841 and 1979.

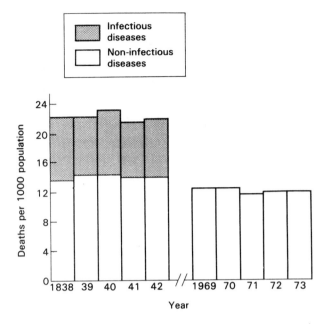

Fig. 9.6 Crude annual death rates from infectious and non-infectious diseases 1838–1842 and 1969–1973. (Death rates from infectious diseases during 1969–1973 were too low to show on this scale.)

(Fig. 9.6). For most of these, mortality rates were highest amongst young people. It is apparent that the virtual disappearance of these diseases from the UK, and from most countries in the Western world, owed more to improvements in the general quality of life and to improvements in public and personal hygiene than they did to any specific medical measures. Specific medical treatments were not introduced until long after the mortality rates from these diseases had undergone the greater part of their fall. It is noteworthy that many of the lethal diseases of nineteenth century Europe are now regarded as 'tropical diseases' and are associated with the type of poverty that is prevalent in some of the under-developed countries of the world. They are more properly called 'poverty diseases'. The principal diseases that accounted for the high mortality and which have now been controlled or eliminated in the Western world were tuberculosis, the enteric fevers, cholera, smallpox, scarlet fever, measles, whooping cough and diphtheria.

During the 1840s about 18% of all deaths were attributed to tuberculosis. It is possible that some of these may have been misdiagnosed carcinoma of the bronchus or some other disease of the respiratory system, but the numbers were so large that there can be little doubt that the downward trend in mortality rates shown in Fig. 3.1 was mainly a reflection of tuberculosis control. The decline in tuberculosis mortality preceded the identification of the organism or any specific treatment. Although the principal explanation for this remarkable trend probably lies in improvements in diet and in consequent enhancement of the resistance of individuals, the practice of isolating cases, thereby reducing the spread of the disease, probably also had an effect.

The enteric and diarrhoeal diseases were endemic in the nineteenth century and were a particularly important cause of death amongst infants and children. Their impact began to decline in the 1870s (Fig. 9.7) and seemed to be the result of improvements in personal hygiene and in child rearing practices. A more specific measure, the provision of a pure water supply, was responsible for the disappearance of cholera as an endemic disease in the British Isles (Fig. 9.8).

Because of the obvious physical signs of smallpox the statistics on its

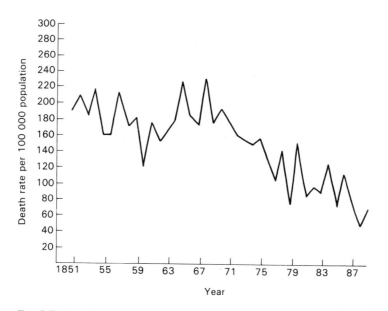

Fig. 9.7 Mortality rates from enteric fevers in England and Wales 1851–1889.

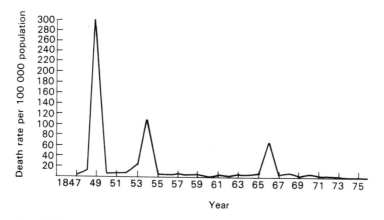

Fig. 9.8 Cholera mortality in England and Wales 1847–1877.

mortality are likely to have been accurate. This disease was endemic in the nineteenth century (Fig. 9.9). Typically there were superimposed regular epidemics every 6–7 years. The frequency of these epidemics was probably due to changes in herd immunity. Contact with disease either resulted in death or lifelong immunity, thereby reducing the size of the susceptible population. Following an epidemic, most survivors would be immune and this decreased the risk to the remaining susceptibles. When the proportion of susceptibles in the population increased (by the birth of children), a further epidemic occurred. Not surprisingly, the majority of deaths occurred amongst children and infants. The elimination of this disease was due to a specific medical measure, the dicovery of vaccination. However, it should be noted that although vaccination became compulsory in 1852, the law was not widely enforced for a further 20 years.

The other infectious diseases that ceased to be a major cause of mortality included scarlet fever which was endemic and had regular superimposed epidemics. Its eventual elimination was probably due mainly to the advent of more successful treatment for the complications of the disease. Measles mortality presents a similar picture (Fig. 9.10). The elimination of diphtheria was probably related to the discovery first of an antitoxin and then of a vaccine.

Clearly the measures that have achieved the control of the infectious diseases

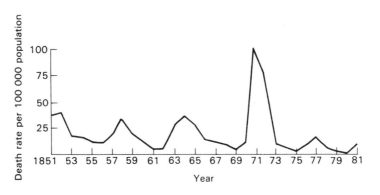

Fig. 9.9 Smallpox mortality in England and Wales 1851–1881.

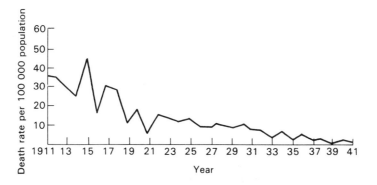

Fig. 9.10 Measles mortality in England and Wales 1911–1941.

are to a large extent byproducts of improvements in the quality of life and, more recently, relatively simple medical measures. All should be applicable, and are being applied in poorer countries of the world at the present time with consequent accelerating reductions in their mortality levels.

Factors affecting fertility in communities

It has been shown that reductions in mortality have been achieved either as byproducts of tangible and universally acceptable improvements in the environment or from certain specific medical measures, such as vaccination, which reduce the risk of contracting diseases. By contrast, reductions in the fertility of a population require the consent and cooperation of individuals together with changes in their personal attitudes to child bearing and child rearing. In pre-transitional populations it is necessary for women to bear large numbers of children in order that there will be sufficient survivors to maintain the size of the community and to provide a work force to sustain essential activities. Strong social customs and belief systems have grown up to support this need and, therefore, changes in fertility depend on changes in social customs and ethics. Next, it is necessary to make the knowledge of fertility control available to the individuals themselves.

Social factors

By convention, child bearing and child rearing outside marriage are discouraged in most societies. In contemporary Western societies this attitude has recently begun to change but in most of the world, powerful taboos remain and societies continue to censure the unmarried mother and her child. Thus marriage practices have a potent effect on the reproductive behaviour of societies.

The legal minimum age of marriage is of less importance in most societies than the conventional age of marriage. It is, however, used as a means of reducing population growth in some countries, notably China, where it has recently been raised by 2 years. Although conception may still take place below the minimum age for marriage, the pregnancy is stigmatized as illegitimate.

The conventional age of marriage tends to be several years greater than the legal minimum. In nineteenth century Sweden the conventional age of marriage was the mid to late twenties. This convention was imposed in rural communities by obliging a man to demonstrate his ability to support his wife before marriage could take place and by his living apart from women during the period he was becoming established. Although the age-specific legitimate fertility rates of Swedish women at this time were close to the maximum possible, the effective duration of the fertile period was reduced. In Ireland there has always been a tendency for late marriage. In England and Wales there have been significant changes in the age of first marriage during the past 70 years (Table 9.2). The effect of the proportion of women who are married on age-specific birth rates is obvious from Table 9.3. The legitimate birth rate to women aged 20–24 was similar in 1939 and 1969 but the age-specific birth rates differ considerably because the proportion of women who were married changes between years.

Divorce, separation and widowhood have the reverse effect on birth rates to

Table 9.2 First marriage rates per 1000 single women in England and Wales. (Source: Registrar General's Annual Statistical Reviews.)

	Age in years		
	16–19	20–24	25–29
1938	28.1	171.6	132.2
1948	49.1	212.5	158.1
1958	75.2	260.8	162.5
1968	84.6	260.9	161.4
1978	58.8	177.9	134.8
1988	23.0	101.6	106.8

Table 9.3 Births to women aged 20–24 years in England and Wales. (Source: Registrar General's Annual Statistical Reviews.)

	Legitimate births per 1000 married women	Percentage of women who were married	Births per 1000 women (married and single)
1939	252	33	93
1969	251	58	157
1988	212	30	95

those of marriage. The same conventions that discourage never-married women from having children discourage divorced and widowed women from reproducing. In normal times this has little impact on birth rates but, following World War I, when many women in Europe were widowed, there was a noticeable reduction in the number of births, although there had been little change in the size of the female population in the reproductive age group.

Sexual behaviour within marriage varies between societies. Although taboos exist regarding the permissibility of intercourse at certain times, e.g. during menstruation or religious feasts, this has little measurable effect on birth rates.

Contraception

Although the possibility of contraception and knowledge of techniques has existed for many years (it was known to and used by the ancient Egyptians) its use varies substantially from place to place depending on its acceptability, availability and efficiency.

Nowadays, in most societies, the most important social factor determining the patterns of reproduction is the acceptability of contraception. This is determined to some extent by religious beliefs. Members of the Roman Catholic Church are forbidden to use artificial methods of birth control. Nevertheless, the rule of the church is not universally adhered to and contraceptive practice varies amongst Roman Catholics. It has been shown that a large proportion of Roman Catholics in Europe and North America no longer adhere to their church's teaching. The better educated (and those who are better off) are more likely to use contraception than the ill-educated and poor.

The Roman Catholic Church is not the only religious group actively to discourage the practice of contraception. Within Christian cultures the Hutterite and Amish communities take the Biblical dictum to go forth and multiply quite literally and amongst them it is not unusual for married women to produce a dozen or more children. Some non-Christian religious groups also eschew contraception on principle.

Local ethics and morals may restrict the availability of the more efficient methods to certain groups. Thus if sexual intercourse outside marriage is deemed wrong, contraception for the unmarried may be seen as a collusion with immorality. Until recently, many clinics in England and some general practitioners would not advise unmarried women on contraception.

In societies where the role of women is seen mainly as child bearing and child rearing, women who limit their fertility may be rejected or may fear rejection. Similar problems affect the acceptability of contraception in groups where a man's success and strength is measured by the number of children he fathers. During transition between high and low mortality, fear of death of existing infants and children, resulting in the extinction of the family, leads to the production of more children. It is often difficult to convince parents in such societies that the survival of existing children is threatened by further enlargement of the family.

Even if the idea of birth control is acceptable to an individual the method of contraception involved may be unacceptable. Many of the simpler methods require action by the male, (e.g. the sheath or coitus interruptus) but they may detract from his satisfaction. The methods that require no action at the time of intercourse usually require intervention by trained professionals, (e.g. the IUD or sterilization). The choice and use of methods of contraception is also affected by the couple's level of education. This is an important factor in communities where birth control is new and where modern techniques are not common knowledge. Most developing countries have recognized this important factor and are experimenting with teaching methods. The most effective methods are usually the most expensive. If family economics mean that people cannot afford the new technology then in practice the method is not available to them. The problem of cost is greatest in countries with the greatest problems.

The efficiency of a particular method of contraception is assessed by the number of conceptions per women-years of use. The assessment should be made on a group similar to that in which the method will be used. Table 9.4 shows estimates of relative efficiency of some of the current methods. These estimates were made in married women who were likely to have regular intercourse and to be motivated to use the method correctly. Some women use contraceptive methods incorrectly. For example, there is some evidence that single women are erratic in their use of oral contraceptives which alters the apparent effectiveness of the method.

Table 9.4 The relative efficiency of different methods of contraception.

Contraceptive used	Pregnancies per 100 women-years of use
Oral contraceptives	0.15
IUD	2.00
Diaphragm	2.40–5.00

In 1969 a great deal of publicity was given to the possible danger of producing venous thrombo-embolic disease by oral contraceptives and a large number of women precipitately stopped using them. They did not appear to use alternative methods and consequently the decline in birth rate in England and Wales was temporarily halted (Fig. 9.11).

Some recent changes in the patterns of fertility in England and Wales

During the past 50 years there has been a tendency for women to marry earlier. The mean interval between first marriage and the birth of the first child fell until the early 1970s when it began to increase (Fig. 9.12). The increase in the interval between first marriage and first pregnancy was associated with an increase in the use of efficient contraception, particularly oral contraception and the IUD. The mean interval between marriage and pregnancy is affected by the proportion of women who are pregnant when they marry. Figure 9.13 shows that in the 1960s, about 40% of women who married under the age of 20 years and about 15% of women aged 20–29 were pregnant when they married. The proportions fell in all age groups during the 1970s. The post 1970s changes were due to a combination of increased availability of abortion and of contraception to unmarried people. This hypothesis is consistent with the fall both in the illegitimate birth rate and the number of marriages of pregnant women.

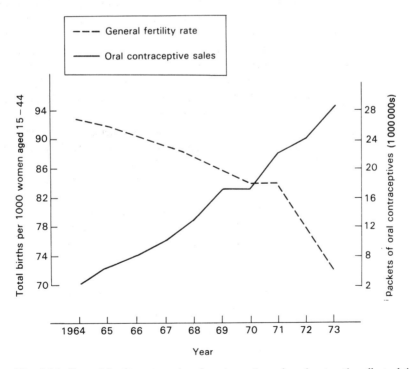

Fig. 9.11 General fertility rate and oral contraceptive sales, showing the effect of the 1969 'pill scare'.

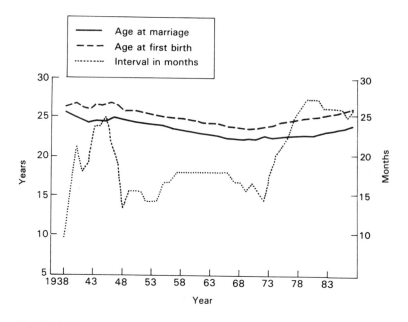

Fig. 9.12 Average age of women at marriage and average age at birth of first legitimate child (England and Wales).

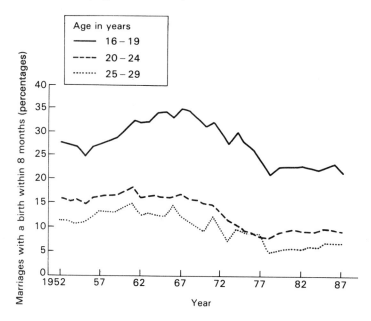

Fig. 9.13 Trends in illegitimate conceptions (England and Wales).

Figure 9.14 shows the cumulative age-specific fertility rates for cohorts of women born in different years. The 1921 and 1931 cohorts reached their peak birth rates at about the age of 26 and fertility was high well into the 30s. By

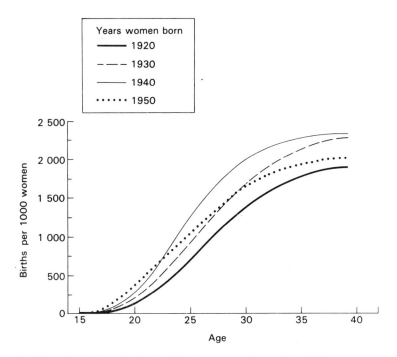

Fig. 9.14 Cumulative fertility of birth cohorts in England and Wales.

contrast, the 1941 cohort reached its peak fertility at age 24 and tended to have more children earlier in their lives. The 1951 cohorts' fertility was stable between the ages of 21 and 28 years. It is probable that family size of the pre 1941 cohorts was determined largely by the age of marriage and that, within marriage, conscious control of fertility was haphazard, whilst the post 1941 cohorts married earlier and exercised a more precise conscious control over fertility.

Fetal loss and infant mortality

Fetal and infant survival rates are amongst the most important factors influencing demographic change. Fetal loss during pregnancy occurs in three ways:

> spontaneous abortion;
> induced abortion;
> still births.

In developed countries 15–25% of known conceptions spontaneously abort, the true rate may be as high as 40% and 60% of spontaneous abortions have abnormal chromosomes. In the process of demographic transition changes in spontaneous abortion and still birth rates are not significant elements. Induced abortion depends upon individual motivation and it affects age-specific birth rates selectively. In countries where induced abortion is legal, full statistics are published. Figure 9.15 shows the numbers of 'known' conceptions in women

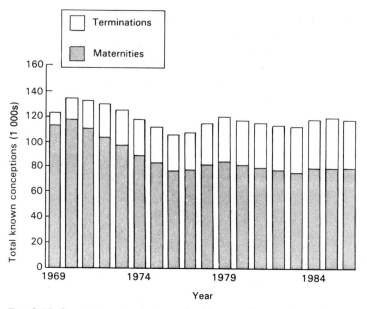

Fig. 9.15 Conceptions in women under 20 years, distinguishing those leading to maternities from those terminated by abortion.

aged 16–19 years in England and Wales from 1969 to 1986 and demonstrates the contribution of legal abortion to the fall in birth rate.

Perinatal and infant mortality rates are sometimes used as sensitive indicators of the quality of health services within a country or within a district. This is asserted because some of the causes of perinatal deaths are avoidable by medical intervention.

There have been three major studies of perinatal deaths in Britain in 1946, 1958 and 1970. Cohorts of births were followed-up beyond the perinatal period to examine factors related to perinatal mortality and morbidity. They showed that adverse maternal obstetric factors act in a cumulative manner.

Perinatal mortality rates (PMR) are highest in multiparous (para 3 plus) women, in women at the end of reproductive life and when the birth interval is less than 12 months or more than 60 months. Conversely they are lowest in para 1 women, women aged 20–19 years and when the birth interval is 18–35 months. The PMR is higher for illegitimate births than it is for legitimate births, even after account is taken of parity and maternal age. There is a positive social class gradient, i.e. social class V has PMR greater than social class I. Some social class differences are due to reproductive behaviour. Birth weight is highly correlated with perinatal mortality—the proportion of the low birth weight babies born within a country largely determines its perinatal mortality rate. Also, there is a close correlation between low birth weight and certain maternal factors, e.g. parity, birth interval and maternal age.

Poor maternal health can also adversely affect perinatal mortality rates. Important diseases or conditions that have been shown to be associated with high PMR include:

hypertension;

poorly controlled diabetes;

renal disease (which can also decrease fertility);

infection (hepatitis B, syphilis, rubella, CMV and toxoplasmosis can cause fetal abnormalities);

severe malnutrition;

smoking;

alcohol can cause fetal alcohol syndrome (intrauterine growth retardation, developmental delay and spontaneous abortion).

Thus, while a large proportion of fetal and perinatal mortality is difficult to prevent, much can be done to reduce rates by appropriate antenatal and postnatal care and advice.

Summary

• Every industrialized nation has low mortality compared with non-industrialized countries. Further substantial decline in mortality in industrialized countries is unlikely because the major causes of death are associated with old age.

• There is great potential for further substantial reduction in mortality in Asia, Africa and Latin America. This will be achieved by control of the major infective diseases, especially gastrointestinal and respiratory infections.

• The principal factors acting against any quick reduction in mortality in developing countries are malnutrition, illiteracy and poverty.

• Industrialization is inversely related to changes in fertility. Four explanations for this can be adduced:

(a) in urban societies children are not an economic asset;

(b) as the infant death rate declines the proportion of children who survive to adulthood increases and the number of births required to attain a desired family size is smaller;

(c) in urban societies there are greater opportunities for women outside the domestic environment and being committed to child rearing restricts a woman's activities;

(d) in educated societies the influence of secular rationality is stronger which allows readier acceptance of contraception.

Definitions

Abortion

Expulsion of the product of conception before it has reached an age when it could be expected to have an independent life and shows no signs of life at birth. The lower limit of fetal viability is defined as 28 weeks gestation.

Still birth

Delivery of a fetus which shows no signs of life after a presumed 28 weeks gestation.

Still birth rate
Still births per thousand *total* births (both live and still).

Perinatal mortality rate
Still births plus deaths within the first week of life per thousand *total* births (both live and still).

Neonatal mortality rate
Deaths of live born infants before the 28th day of life per thousand live births.

Infant mortality rate
Deaths of children under 1 year, i.e. infants per thousand live births.

Part 2
Prevention and Control of Disease

Chapter 10
General Principles

Introduction

Until recent times people tended to accept ill-health and even premature death as unavoidable hazards of human existence. Now, however, they have come to expect to live long and healthy lives. If illness occurs it is assumed that modern medicine can, or ought to be able to, restore the sufferer to full normal activity. These changed expectations have been brought about to a large extent by the publicity given to some of the more dramatic advances in medical knowledge and treatments and by evident success in reducing mortality, particularly during infancy and childhood. It is, of course, true that during the past fifty or so years the scope of medical treatments has been extended greatly. They are now more specific than hitherto and their results have been improved. However, it is also true that most of the diseases which commonly affect man are self-limiting and that medical treatment does little to alter their natural course. Furthermore, of the diseases that result in death or major disability, relatively few can be cured. The main impact of modern medicine has tended to be to allow people to live longer and more comfortably with their diseases rather than to die from them or be incapacitated by them. Members of the public often fail to appreciate these facts. The corollary is that for many of the major diseases it is both logical and desirable to take steps to prevent their occurrence. Moreover, even if a treatment eventually becomes available, a strategy of prevention would do more to reduce human suffering. In future, therefore, it is likely that medical research and practice will be expected to give greater attention to the means whereby health can be promoted and diseases prevented. For some diseases this is already possible and the prospects for further advances in this direction are improving.

In the past, infectious diseases were the major causes of morbidity and mortality, particularly in children and young adults, in the Western world. It has already been pointed out that their control over the past 150 years owes more to social and economic progress than it does to specific medical intervention. Preventive programmes during this period have included such measures as improvements in sanitation, water supply, the quantity and quality of food, the quality of housing, conditions in the workplace and raised standards of personal hygiene. All of these carried obvious and immediate benefits other than those purely related to health: they made life more comfortable and pleasant with little or no restriction on personal freedom. In fact most of the changes were at community level and were brought about by legislation rather than requiring action by individuals, which made them comparatively easy to institute.

By contrast, some of the more recent advances in the control and prevention of communicable diseases such as the elimination of diphtheria and poliomyelitis in many countries and the world-wide eradication of smallpox, required mainly medical action (immunization) and thus can rightly be claimed as major medical achievements. The benefits of environmental improvements, as well as of specific immunization, however, will be sustained only by continued vigilance and much modern preventive medicine is still directed to this end. In the past, the presence of a disease in the community served as a constant reminder of its nature and consequences. In societies dependent upon distant memories of serious infectious illness in childhood and once common lethal infections such as cholera, typhoid and tuberculosis, continued public education is essential to maintain the present position.

The virtual elimination of the older life-threatening infectious diseases has brought the non-infectious illnesses into greater prominence. In modern times despite the emergence of new infectious disease threats such as Legionnaires disease and HIV infection, it is malignancies, degenerative conditions (such as arthritis), cardiovascular disease and, other chronic illnesses that occur amongst older people that are the major problems. For most of these the available treatments are as unsatisfactory as were the treatments for infectious diseases in the nineteenth century. However, their prevention is more complicated and progress is more difficult to achieve.

The problems centre around the natural history of the diseases themselves. Generally these diseases are characterized by having a long latent period between exposure to the aetiological agent or environment and the appearance of symptoms. In many cases the symptoms have an insidious onset and by the time they are of sufficient severity to cause the affected individual to seek medical attention, irreparable damage has been done. Prevention moreover often depends on actions by the individual, rather than passively enjoying improvements in the quality of life brought about by the actions of others. It demands modification of behaviour in such matters as the use of tobacco and alcohol, diet, exercise, etc. at a time in life when the risks of contracting the disease in question are seen as remote. It is also a fact that, even for common diseases, the absolute risks for the individual are indeed relatively small. In these circumstances campaigns to persuade people to change their lifestyle require great skill and patience applied over long periods of time. Public policies in such matters as the taxation of tobacco and alcohol products, the subsidizing of food production, e.g. EEC dairy subsidies, and public provision of recreational facilities, also have major health implications and changes require a political will to be implemented. Despite these obvious and real difficulties, prevention remains an important aspiration and progress is being made in some of these diseases, e.g. in reduction of cancer mortality, both by action at a political and community level and by persuading people to change their lifestyle and habits.

Principles of prevention

Disease is a result of a harmful interaction between the *host* (man), the pathogenic *agent* and the *environment* (Fig. 10.1). Agent, host and environment form a dynamic system in which, in the healthy individual, the balance normally favours the host. This is the case if the agent is locally absent or contained, or its capacity to cause disease is matched by man's protective

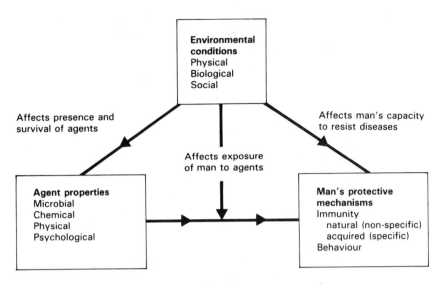

Fig. 10.1 Interactions of agent, host and environment, causing disease.

mechanisms, or the environment inhibits the spread of the agent. Disease or injury occurs when the balance is disturbed, e.g. owing to changes in the pathogenicity of an agent, changes in environmental conditions that favour the survival and transmission of the agent to man, or the breakdown or absence of man's normal defence mechanisms. Conversely, the control and prevention of disease depends on effective intervention in the relationship between agent, host and environment to ensure that the balance remains in man's favour, or, if disease does occur, to ensure that its progress is rapidly arrested or reversed or its consequences minimized.

Useful preventive action does not necessarily require knowledge of aetiology and many examples of effective prevention that preceded complete understanding of cause could be cited. For example, in the eighteenth century Lind demonstrated that during long sea voyages scurvy in the crews of ships could be prevented by the consumption of adequate amounts of fresh fruit; this was long before vitamin C was discovered. In the nineteenth century John Snow showed that cholera was transmitted by drinking water polluted by sewage. His findings led to the elimination of cholera by the provision of a pure water supply many decades before the isolation of the causal organism. In this century Doll and Hill (see Chapters 5 and 6) demonstrated that those who stop smoking cigarettes, substantially reduce their risk of contracting lung cancer, though the carcinogenic agent in tobacco smoke has yet to be identified. In general, however, a full and accurate understanding of the causes of diseases and of the factors that determine the balance between agent, host and environment is helpful in order to construct appropriately directed preventive and control programmes. Epidemiological studies are used to identify the agents and those elements in the environment or in people's behaviour and personal characteristics which are key determinants of the natural history of disease.

Intervention strategies

Three main types of intervention strategy are possible, based on this knowledge:

strategy related to the agent;

strategy related to the environment;

strategy related to man.

Strategy related to the agent

If the agent can be identified it may be possible to remove or destroy it at source. For example, the incidence of pneumoconiosis in coal miners was reduced by dust control in the mines; the control of bovine tuberculosis was achieved by eradication of the disease from milking herds.

Strategy related to the environment

This includes attention to general environmental factors such as standards of housing, nutrition, working conditions, water supplies, sewage disposal and the control of environmental pollution. Environmental measures specifically related to individual diseases are also important. People may be protected from potentially injurious agents by the construction of barriers between them and the source of harm. For example, the use of machine guards in industry reduces the risk of accidents occurring; the transmission of foodborne infection is prevented by hygienic food production methods: animal or insect vectors may be dealt with as in action to prevent the spread of malaria or yellow fever by mosquito control.

Strategy related to man

There are three different strategies involving individuals.

1   The enhancement of general or specific resistance to disease, e.g. by improved nutrition or immunization.

2   The modification of personal behaviour, e.g. by persuading people to adopt healthier life styles by not smoking, moderating alcohol intake, improving diet, avoiding obesity, exercising regularly, etc.

3   The use of screening to detect predisposing conditions or the early stages of disease when action can be taken to prevent its onset or control its progress, e.g. tuberculin testing for tuberculosis or blood pressure measurement to identify hypertension, mammography for breast cancer detection.

Preventive action

Action is also sometimes classified as:

primary prevention;

secondary prevention;

tertiary prevention.

Primary prevention

This is aimed at preventing the disease process from starting. Most strategies are directed to the removal or destruction of agents. Environmental control, as well as immunization, health education and nutritional advice fall into this category.

Secondary prevention

This aims to detect disease at the earliest possible stage and to institute measures to prevent its further progression. Screening programmes are the most important examples of secondary prevention.

Tertiary prevention

This aims at 'damage limitation' in persons with manifest disease by modifying continuing risk factors such as smoking and the implementation of effective programmes of rehabilitation.

Where a choice of strategy exists, the planning of a preventive programme should take account of certain practical considerations. The most desirable approach is the one giving the greatest benefit to the largest number of people. Action which is simple and requires minimal cooperation from individuals is usually the most successful. Economic considerations should not be neglected when deciding on a particular course of action.

For convenience, strategies for prevention are considered under the following general headings:
- Prevention directed to environmental action:
  agents and environmental control;
  occupational health and accidents.
- Prevention directed to personal action:
  immunization;
  health education and nutrition;
  screening.

The distinction between environmental and personal action is often blurred and it is not possible to separate the two completely.

Chapter 11
Agents and Environmental Control

Introduction

Strategies for control and prevention of diseases caused by infection or noxious physical agents are usually either based on action directed at the agent itself (at source or during transmission to the human host) or on enhancing the immunity of those at risk of exposure. The design of a rational and effective programme requires a clear understanding of the relationship between the agent, the environment and man in each particular instance. Account must be taken of the properties of the agent which affect its ability to survive and cause disease, the ways in which individual and population immunity operates, and how the environment can affect the balance between the two directly and indirectly. Therefore, this chapter begins with an account of the main factors involved in such ecological systems.

AGENTS

Pathogenic agents

A pathogenic agent is any living organism, chemical substance, physical phenomenon, e.g. ionizing radiation, or other environmental circumstance which acts directly on man to cause disease. In some diseases a single agent is involved, e.g. microbes in infectious diseases, in others several agents may act either synergistically, e.g. asbestos exposure and cigarette smoking in lung cancer, or independently, e.g. ionizing radiation and chemical carcinogens in some other forms of cancer.

Pathogenic agents can be classified as :
inanimate agents;
biological agents.

Inanimate agents

These may be exogenous or endogenous to the host.

Exogenous agents

A wide range of potentially noxious substances may be found in the air, in food, in water and other environmental situations, e.g. poisons used in industrial processes, allergens (such as pollen), drugs, exhaust fumes, tobacco smoke and chemicals used as food preservatives. In addition excessive heat or cold, radiation and other factors may result in disease.

Endogenous agents

Abnormal products of metabolism or accumulation of products caused by defective mechanisms for their breakdown or excretion can produce disease, e.g. uraemia in kidney failure.

The type of damage caused by non-biological agents is largely determined by their route of entry and the dose. Damage may be structural, cellular or biochemical.

Biological agents (micro-organisms)

These can be bacteria, viruses or parasites. The majority of microbes are harmless to man. Some, although not universally pathogenic, are potentially dangerous and may cause disease in unusual circumstances. Caution is needed in attributing a disease to an organism which fortuitously happens to be present.

There are many factors that determine whether or not biological agents cause disease in any particular situation. They can be broadly divided into host-related biological factors, intrinsic properties of organisms and the presence of reservoirs of infection.

Host-related biological properties

Infectivity

The infectivity of an organism is its capacity to multiply in or on the tissue of the host. This varies between microbial species, between individuals and with the route of entry. It may also be affected by the presence of tissue trauma which facilitates the entry of organisms and provides a suitable growth medium.

Pathogenicity

The pathogenicity of an organism is its capacity to cause disease in an infected host, i.e. number of cases of disease/total persons infected. In the days before smallpox was eradicated nearly every infection with smallpox virus in susceptible persons caused disease (high pathogenicity) whereas many people infected with polio virus are asymptomatic (low pathogenicity).

Virulence

Virulence is the pathogenicity of an organism in a specific host. Different strains of the same agent may vary in virulence, e.g. 'wild' strains of measles and polio virus are virulent in man in contrast to the attenuated strains used in vaccines. Likewise some strains of Corynebacterium diphtheriae produce toxin and therefore cause disease while others are non-toxogenic and therefore non-pathogenic. The virulence of particular organisms may vary over time, the virulence of the streptococcus for example appears to have diminished over the last 50 years.

Immunogenicity

Immunogenicity is the capacity of an organism to induce specific and lasting immunity in the host. Some organisms are antigenically more potent than others. Those that invade the blood stream, e.g. measles virus, are more likely to produce a good immune response than those organisms that only infect surface membranes, e.g. the gonococcus.

Intrinsic properties of organisms

Physical dimensions and chemical structure

The physical dimensions and chemical structure of agents may be important in certain circumstances, e.g. difference in size between viruses, bacteria and parasites. Two agents with similar structures may stimulate a similar immune response which confers mutual protection, e.g. the use of vaccinia virus to immunize against smallpox.

Growth requirements

Some organisms are more fastidious in their growth requirements than others, e.g. viruses can only replicate within living cells whereas enterobacteria can grow in media with minimal nutrient content.

Survival

Organisms vary in their capacity to survive in the free state and to withstand adverse environmental conditions, e.g. heat, cold, dryness. Spore-forming organisms, such as tetanus bacilli which can survive for years in a dormant state, have a major advantage over an organism like the gonococcus which survives for a very short time outside the human host.

Life cycle

The life cycle of certain organisms have important consequences on the spread of disease. Organisms such as the malaria parasite which have a complex life cycle requiring a vector are more vulnerable than those with simpler requirements for transmission. In many infections by such organisms man is an accidental host.

Host specificity

Some organisms, such as the tubercle bacillus and brucella, can infect many species of animal, in contrast to smallpox or measles viruses which infect only man. Flexibility in choice of host is clearly to the agent's advantage.

Antigenically stable organisms

Organisms which are antigenically stable or exist in only one antigenic form, e.g. measles virus, usually induce lifelong immunity. If the agent is unstable, e.g. influenza virus, or exists in many antigenic forms, e.g. rhinovirus, man cannot develop lasting immunity. Environmental conditions, such as those created by the indiscriminate use of antimicrobial drugs, may select out the more virulent and resistant strains of bacteria from among several co-existing variants.

Reservoirs of infection

A reservoir of infection is the site or sites in which a microbe normally lives and reproduces. Reservoirs of infection may be classified as human and other biological or environmental.

Human reservoirs

In some infectious diseases such as many respiratory virus diseases, the patient sheds virulent organisms in large quantities during the acute phase of illness. This results in risk to contacts. Sub-clinical infections may be as dangerous as infections in obviously sick people and often account for cases that have no clear link with others.

Carriers

Carriers are of three types:
  healthy;
  convalescent;
  chronic.
Healthy carriers are persons who are colonized by the organism without any detectable reaction, e.g. staphylococcal carriage in the anterior nares or in the axilla. Convalescent carriers are persons who have recovered from the illness but who continue temporarily to excrete the organism, e.g. salmonellae in faeces. Chronic carriers are persons who, while remaining clinically well, may carry and excrete organisms continuously or intermittently over a prolonged period, e.g. typhoid carriers in whom S. typhi may remain in the gallbladder for life. Such carriers are a continuing threat to the community long after disease has been controlled.

Other biological or environmental reservoirs

The link between man and reservoirs of infection in his environment is not always clear. Methods of transmission can include eating and drinking infected foodstuffs, e.g. salmonellae from poultry or brucella from milk; contact with sick animals, e.g. rabies, psittacosis; handling biological products, e.g. anthrax from wool and hides, Q fever from sheep placenta; contact with animals which harbour vectors, e.g. typhus, plague; direct inoculation by arthropods, e.g. malaria, arboviruses.

Host factors

The occurrence of disease in man depends on his susceptibility to the agents to which he is exposed. His defence mechanisms are:
  natural immunity (non-specific);
  acquired (specific) immunity;
  population (herd) immunity.

Natural immunity

Some individuals appear to have an exceptional susceptibility to disease which is probably inherited. This can be seen in the similar susceptibility of monozygotic twins and different susceptibility of dizygotic twins to certain diseases. In national or ethnic groups natural selection over many generations may eventually breed a relatively resistant stock. A good example of this phenomenon is the history of tuberculosis in Europe. Over the last century or more the population has experienced a high incidence of this disease which, by causing high mortality amongst susceptible young adults tended to favour the survival through reproductive life of those with higher innate resistance. By contrast when an infectious disease is introduced into a community with no recent experience of it the result can be disastrous, e.g. the introduction of measles to the Greenland Eskimos by the American forces during World War II caused devastating epidemics.

There is some evidence that the two sexes have different susceptibilities to specific diseases. In general, males experience higher mortality rates than females for most diseases, although the incidence is often higher in females. This apparent difference may relate more to life style, e.g. occupation, and exposure to particular hazards, e.g. contact with children than to inherent differences in immunity.

The body has a wide tolerance for variation in nutritional intake. However, large excesses or gross prolonged deficiencies are harmful. Malnutrition increases the severity of infectious diseases, such as measles, while breast feeding probably shelters the infant from the risk of gastrointestinal infections.

Acquired (specific) immunity

Specific immunity to infection is usually mediated through the presence of antibodies in the blood, tissue fluids and secretions. They may be naturally or artificially acquired, and in either case the acquistion may be active or passive.

- *Natural active immunity* is acquired by natural infection with the agent which produces either clinical illness or inapparent infection.
- *Natural passive immunity*. Antibodies in the maternal blood are transmitted across the placenta to the fetus and persist in the newborn infant for some months.
- *Artificial active immunity* is induced by the administration of vaccines, which contain the relevant antigen in a harmless form.
- *Artificial passive immunity*. After exposure to potentially dangerous infections, e.g. tetanus, diphtheria or rabies, blood products containing antibodies (human or animal serum or immunoglobulin) are sometimes used to provide temporary protection.

Population (herd) immunity

The resistance of groups of people to spread of infection is termed population (or herd) immunity. It depends on the proportion of individuals in the population who are immune. If this is sufficiently high, chains of transmission of the agent cannot be sustained because susceptible persons in the group are shielded from exposure to infected persons by the immune persons around them. The degree of herd immunity which will inhibit spread varies with different infections but is less than 100%. It depends on:

- the frequency of new introductions of infection;

- the degree of mixing which affects opportunities for contact between infected and susceptible persons;
- the transmissibility of the infection and duration of infectiousness of excreters. Herd immunity affects the periodicity of epidemics. So long as each case leads to more than one new infection, the incidence of the disease increases and herd immunity rises. When herd immunity reaches a level at which each case causes less than one new infection, incidence declines. As individual immunity wanes or susceptibles are introduced to the group, herd immunity again declines and the group is again vulnerable. This pattern is well illustrated by the periodic epidemics of measles which occurred before vaccination was introduced (see Fig. 3.4, p. 18). If the antigenic composition of the agent changes or if an agent previously absent from the population is introduced, the benefits of herd immunity are absent and large scale epidemics may result. For example, the periodic antigenic changes of the influenza virus lead to world wide pandemics from time to time.

The environment and disease

The environment is the physical, biological and social world external to the individual. Factors in the environment which directly or indirectly affect health can be divided into:

physical and biological;

social.

Physical and biological environment

Climate

This regulates the natural flora and fauna and the parasites that can survive and be transmitted. For example, if the ambient temperature is warm, the multiplication of salmonellae in contaminated food is accelerated; malaria is transmitted only where the climate favours survival of anopheles mosquitoes. In addition, climate affects certain human activities, such as sport, type of clothing worn, housing and occupation, which in turn affect the probability of exposure to agents of disease.

Geological conditions

These prescribe the routes and ease of communications between communities and consequently the speed with which infective agents can spread. Infection which spreads from person to person does so more rapidly where there is overcrowding, whether in slum tenements or village communal huts.

Man-made conditions

These can mitigate the effects of many adverse external conditions, e.g. central heating and air conditioning. However, in modifying his environment, man often creates new hazards, e.g. air and water pollution, noise, exposure to radiation from nuclear fission, chemical preservatives in food, etc.

Occupations

The occupations followed by people in industrialized societies are associated with a variety of specific hazards from the processes employed, e.g. dust, chemicals, radiation, as well as more subtle influences, e.g. the monotony of machine operations, the stresses of management, etc.

Social environment

In many respects highly developed societies provide a safer environment than those that are less developed. This comes about partly through better environmental sanitation; good housing, clean air, and other physical conditions. Moreover, better education and the provision of better personal and preventive health services lead to an awareness of the importance of a healthy lifestyle. However, economic development also involves industrialization and urbanization. The consequences of these go beyond possible damage to the physical environment. They may lead to disruption of old cultures, weakening of family ties, and the creation of communities where support for the less competent members has to be provided by social welfare services rather than through an integrated community.

Within any society the poorest tend to be least healthy. The consequences of poverty such as poor standards of nutrition, housing, medical services and education, favour high disease rates. The converse also applies; those who suffer from disease, such as the physically and mentally handicapped and those with chronic ailments, have the least earning capacity. Persistent disease in an individual often leads to the phenomenon of downward 'social class migration' since the individual is unable to retain the more demanding types of job and is thus forced to live in progressively poorer circumstances in which he is exposed to greater environmental hazards and risks of disease. This can give a further downward twist in a cycle of deprivation. Contrary to hopes and expectations, since the inception of the NHS there is little sign that the inequalities in health status between social groups in Britain is decreasing. Indeed in some cases they may be increasing. The facts were documented in a report *Inequalities in Health* (the Black Report) published by HMSO in 1980. The report drew attention to the link between these persistent inequalities and the socioeconomic factors influencing the material condition of life of poorer groups, especially children. Its findings were reviewed, updated and substantially confirmed by Whitehead in *The Health Divide*, published by the Health Education Council in 1987.

ENVIRONMENTAL CONTROL

Prevention by specific measures of environmental control

Prevention of disease by measures to control specific aspects of the environment are considered here under the following headings:

    food hygiene;

    the quality of water supplies;

    sewage and waste disposal;

    air pollution control.

Food hygiene

Food poisoning may be caused by either micro-organisms or chemicals. In the case of microbiological food poisoning, the food may be either the vehicle whereby an agent is transmitted or the growth medium for the organisms. For example:

Food as a vehicle

Salmonellosis may be caused by the organism being transmitted from poultry to man in eggs.

Food as a growth medium

During preparation food may become infected with *Staphylococci* from a septic lesion in the food handler. If the food is then stored for long enough at a temperature which allows the organism to multiply, the toxins produced may result in severe symptoms of food poisoning in individuals who consume it. Likewise, improperly stored food may permit the multiplication of *Salmonellae*, *Clostridia* or other pathogens.

The harmful effects of chemicals may arise either from accidental contamination or by the deliberate addition of chemicals to food as preservatives or in order to improve its taste or appearance.

Sources of contamination

Food may become polluted or infected at any stage during its production, manufacture and processing, distribution and preparation for consumption.

Production

Example

Salmonellosis usually owes its origin to the infection of livestock through their food or by cross-infection within herds or poultry flocks. An outbreak of mercury poisoning occurred amongst the residents of Minamata Bay in Japan due to the consumption of fish taken from waters polluted with mercury by industrial effluent.

Manufacture and processing

Example

In 1964 an outbreak of typhoid in Aberdeen was caused by corned beef which had probably become contaminated by use of polluted water to cool cans which had defective seals. The 'Epping Jaundice' outbreak in 1965 was the result of eating bread and cakes that were made from a sack of flour that had been chemically contaminated during transit. The mass production line techniques used in the processing of broiler chickens favour the spread of bacteria such as sallmonellae within the plant. Thus cleanliness in the plant is essential.

Storage and distribution

Example
Outbreaks of food poisoning due to a variety of agents have occurred because butchers, dairies and ice-cream vendors have paid insufficient attention to hygiene when storing and selling their products.

Preparation for consumption

Example
In domestic households and in catering establishments, poor technique, particularly in relation to avoiding contact between raw and cooked meats, inadequate thawing of frozen foods, insufficient cooking and the subsequent careful control of temperature during storage and serving, together with inadequate attention to cleanliness of premises and equipment may lead to food poisoning, such as that due to *Clostridium perfringens*, staphylococcal toxins, or salmonellae.

Prevention of foodborne disease

The prevention of foodborne disease depends on correct action by many individuals in the complex chain of production, manufacture and distribution. The main ways in which the safety of food is maintained and good hygienic practice encouraged are as follows:

Quality of products

There are strict regulations relating to the quality and composition of some foods. This applies particularly to milk and milk products, meat and meat products, shellfish and the use of food additives by manufacturers. Recent concerns relating to the safety of poultry and eggs, certain types of cheese, and of chilled dishes prepared for subsequent reheating have led to much public anxiety and calls for tightening of statutory controls.

Environmental conditions

Environmental Health Officers of local authorities have extensive powers to inspect all food premises and to sample foods. If necessary they can prevent their sale. The Food and Drugs Act (1955) and other relevant legislation laid down standards on the construction and cleanliness of food premises and equipment, and on facilities for the storage and protection of food from contamination.

Education of food handlers

However strict the law, the avoidance of food poisoning depends heavily on those who prepare it. They should understand the importance of such matters as personal and kitchen hygiene in the avoidance of contamination or cross-contamination of foods. They should also appreciate the need, for example, to store food in protected containers and to adequately defrost frozen meat and poultry before cooking. The dangers of incubating organisms, especially in made-up meat dishes; and the importance of refrigeration of foods liable to contamination in order to reduce bacterial growth and of the separation of raw meat from foods to be consumed without further cooking must also be constantly stressed.

Cases of suspected food poisoning should be notified to the Medical Officer for Environmental Health (MOEH) to the local authority who, with the assistance of the Environmental Health Officers, is responsible for their investigation. Outbreaks and single cases of serious infections, such as typhoid, call for immediate investigation and control measures. The results may call for amendment of food production practices in the establishments concerned to avoid the danger of further episodes. National and local arrangements in this field are currently under review following the recommendations of a committee of enquiry into the future development of the public health function (the Acheson Report).

The quality of water supplies

Adequate and safe water supplies are essential to health. To be safe, drinking water must be free from contamination with both pathogenic micro-organisms and harmful chemicals. The main infections spread particularly by water are cholera, typhoid and dysentery. These are derived from the contamination of supplies by human excreta. In countries with modern systems of sewage disposal and domestic water supply, spread by this route is rare and in the case of cholera, virtually unknown. Other infections such as cryptosporidiosis may, however, evade the methods of filtration and chemical treatment which have been successful in controlling cholera, typhoid and dysentery. Chemical pollution may arise from the discharge of effluents from factories into rivers and streams and also from the use of pesticides and fertilizers by farmers in water catchment areas.

In recent years evidence that there is a higher incidence of cardiovascular disease in soft water areas than in hard water areas has accumulated, although a causal relationship has not been established.

The *prevention of waterborne* disease rests on the purification and protection of supplies.

Purification

Storage assists the purification of water by sedimentation of suspended matter and by biological action. It is further purified by filtration through sand or chemical filters. Finally it is sterilized by chlorination which oxidizes organic matter and kills any remaining micro-organisms. The dose of chlorine is controlled in order to maintain a small residual amount of free chlorine in the public supply. The water is then distributed through a closed system of pipes and service reservoirs. Its purity is monitored by regular sampling at various points in the distribution system.

Fluoridation

Where the natural fluoride content of water is high the prevalence of dental caries is substantially less than in low fluoride areas. Controlled experiments have shown that this natural benefit can be obtained by artificial fluoridation of water supplies to a level of 1 ppm (parts per million). Maximum protection is achieved when fluoridated water is consumed throughout the years of tooth development and this benefit is maintained into adult life. Objections have been raised to the practice of fluoridation of public water supplies on the grounds that it is an invasion of individual liberty and that it has potential dangers. However, trials have failed to show that at the recommended levels any harm results. Relatively few water authorities fluoridate their supplies but the practice is now actively encouraged by the health departments in Britain.

Sewage and wastage disposal

The provision of an efficient sewage and waste disposal system was the single most important public health measure taken in the nineteenth century. Although this is now taken for granted it remains central to the protection of food and water supplies, as well as to maintenance of a clean and safe environment.

Sewage treatment

In modern sewage treatment plants, after separation of solids by filtering and sedimentation, the liquid sewage is purified by biological oxidation. The final effluent, which is both clean and safe, is usually discharged into rivers, often to be withdrawn further downstream for water supplies. Unfortunately, some seaside towns still discharge raw sewage into the sea, sometimes even above low-tide level. This practice, although it may not be dangerous, leads to offensive pollution of beaches. Where there is no public sewage disposal system, for example in remote rural areas and on camp-sites, excreta are disposed of by using chemical toilets or septic tanks.

Industrial waste

Special arrangements must be made for the disposal of effluents containing dangerous chemicals or radioactive material. However, much industrial waste still finds its way into rivers and streams. Some are so polluted that fish cannot survive, although this situation is slowly improving.

Air pollution control

Air pollution in industrial areas arises mainly from the combustion of hydrocarbon fuels, i.e. coal and oil. The nature of the pollutants generated is dependent on the fuel being used and the conditions of its combustion.

Industrial furnaces

Grit and dust particles emitted by industrial furnaces fall close to their source. Pollutants from burning of coal and its products and of oil in industrial or domestic fires, and the gases from fuel oil combustion in motor vehicles comprise mainly carbon, sulphur dioxide, nitrogen oxides, carbon monoxide and lead. These substances are distributed widely into the atmosphere. The extent of their dispersal depends on the wind, rainfall and the turbulence created by temperature gradients.

Weather conditions

Occasionally weather conditions arise in which there is temperature inversion, that is a warm air blanket covering a layer of cold air at ground level. In cities this leads to the trapping and rapid accumulation of pollutants known as 'smog'. The acute effects of such high concentrations of pollutants are seen mainly in persons who have pre-existing chronic cardiac or respiratory disease.

Long-term damage to health

The long-term damage to health created by air pollution is difficult to separate from the harmful effects of other factors such as smoking, but acute and chronic chest illnesses are more common in children and in older people living in areas with persistently high levels of pollution.

Example

A dramatic example of the acute effects of air pollution was the historic 'smog' in London in December 1952 (Fig. 11.1) when it was estimated that the fog was responsible for the deaths of 3 500–4 000 people. This led directly to the

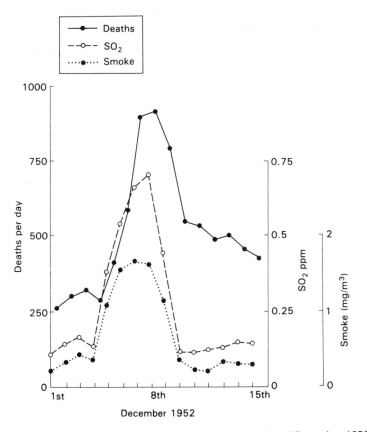

Fig. 11.1 Death and pollution levels in the London fog of December 1952. (Source : *Rep. Public Health Med Subj* **95**; HMSO, London, 1954.)

passing of the Clean Air Act (1956). This Act empowered local authorities to establish smoke control areas. As a result, air pollution by smoke declined rapidly in Britain (Fig. 11.2). The benefit was seen when, in December 1962, London again experienced atmospheric conditions similar to those in 1952 (temperature inversion). The excess number of deaths on this occasion was only about 700. More recently, the contribution of the burning of fossil fuels especially in power stations, to the phenomenon of 'acid rain' with its destructive effects on the forests of central and northern Europe, has been highlighted. This and the damage to the earth's ozone layer caused by the use of chlorofluocarbons (CFCs) as propellants in aerosols and as coolants in refrigerators and freezers have become matters of grave concern to ecologists.

Pollution from vehicles

Pollution from the exhaust of motor vehicles can also be a hazard. Photochemical smog from the emission of hydrocarbons is a major problem in some cities in the USA and Japan. There is increasing pressure for action to abate this source of pollution. Most fuels can be burnt without the emission of smoke but

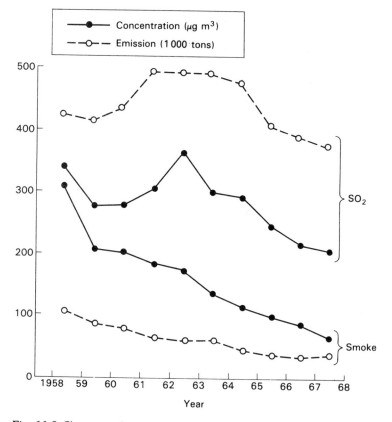

Fig. 11.2 Changes in the emission of smoke and sulphur dioxide and their concentrations in London air (1958–1968).

the control of harmful waste gases is more difficult and is the subject of much discussion and research.

The emission in vehicle exhausts of lead added to petrol to improve its combustion properties has also been condemned for its toxic properties particularly in affecting the cerebral function of children. Although the importance of the contribution of lead in petrol to total environmental exposure to the metal is questioned by some, the process of eliminating lead as a fuel additive is now well under way.

EPIDEMICS/OUTBREAKS

Introduction

The essential characteristic of an epidemic is that it involves a temporary increase in the incidence of a disease, usually circumscribed both in its location and in respect of the groups affected. Rarely it may be *pandemic*, that is have a world-wide distribution. The term *outbreak* is often used to refer to the localized temporary increased incidence of a particular disease. As few as two cases of a disease, associated in time and place, in circumstances where the disease is not a usual occurrence and/or present a particular threat are sufficient to constitute an 'outbreak' requiring investigation, e.g. one or two cases of poliomyelitis.

The pattern of an epidemic depends on the biological properties of the agent, whether or not the environment is favourable to its survival and transmission, and on the immunity of the host population. The course of an epidemic is, therefore, a reflection of time, place and person interaction. Its investigation is an exercise in descriptive epidemiology. Epidemics are usually due to microbial agents although they can arise from other causes such as chemical poisoning.

Definitions

Before describing the nature of epidemics and outbreaks and their investigation it is necessary to explain some of the terms used (Fig. 11.3).

Primary case
This is the first case (or group of cases) arising from the introduction of an agent into a community.

Index case
This term is also used to refer to the initial case.

Secondary cases
Persons who acquire infection from the primary/index case(s) are called secondary cases.

Incubation period
This is the interval between infection of an individual and the onset of symptoms. This differs according to the organism and may vary according to such factors

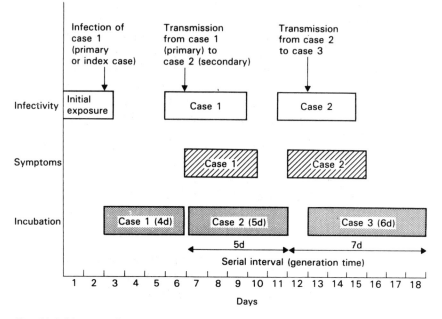

Fig. 11.3 How an infectious disease is transmitted.

as the virulence of the particular strain of the infecting organism, the infecting dose and the susceptibility of the host.

Serial interval/generation time
This is the interval between the onset of primary and secondary cases. This interval may be shorter or longer than the incubation period depending on the duration of infectivity of the primary case, which may start well before and continue for sometime after, the onset of symptoms. When infection in intermediate cases is subclinical, the serial interval may appear to be prolonged.

Derived infection
This is one arising by direct transmission from an infected contact.

Secondary attack rate
This is the number of new cases of a disease arising within one incubation period after the primary case(s):

$$\frac{\text{Number of derived infections}}{\text{Number of susceptible persons in the group at risk}}$$

Types of epidemic
There are two main types of epidemic:
common source;
propagated.

Common source

These epidemics result from the exposure of a group of persons to the same source of infection or noxious substance. If exposure is simultaneous for all subjects, an explosive outbreak will occur one incubation period later and the duration of the epidemic will depend upon individual variation in the range of incubation periods for the disease. Continuous or intermittent exposure of the population to the causal agent produces a more extended and irregular epidemic curve. The control of such outbreaks depends on the early detection of the cause and its removal at source.

Example
An example of an explosive common source outbreak was the epidemic of typhoid in the Swiss skiing resort of Zermatt in 1963 (Fig. 11.4). The vehicle by which *Salmonella typhi* was transmitted in this instance was the mains water supply, one source of which became contaminated.

Common source epidemics have a geographical dimension as well as a time dimension. Cases are most dense around the prime source, e.g. a factory emitting pollution, or concentrated along the lines of distribution of the vehicle, e.g. water or food supply.

Example
An example of this is provided by an outbreak of *Salmonella typhimurium* caused by contaminated salami sticks. The outbreak affected 101 people

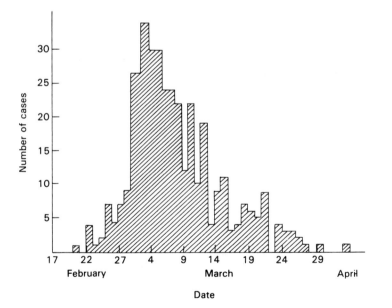

Fig. 11.4 Zermatt typhoid outbreak, 1963: number of cases by date of onset. (Source : Bernard R P. The Zermatt typhoid outbreak in 1963. *J Hyg* (Camb) 1965; **63**, 537.)

between December 1987 and January 1988. It was found that the majority of cases occurred in the south east regions of England (Fig. 11.5) where the product was mainly marketed. A small German salami stick was identified as the source of infection and the product was rapidly withdrawn from sale.

Propagated epidemics

These are due to direct or indirect transmission of the disease from an infected individual person to a susceptible contact. In such cases the epidemic curve usually shows a gradual rise and decline, often with further waves as each successive generation of cases infects a new generation.

The speed at which a propagated outbreak spreads depends on the interaction of a number of factors. These include the opportunity for contact between infected and susceptible persons which is itself influenced both by the density of population and by the level of herd immunity. Obviously person to person epidemics are more likely to occur where large numbers of susceptible persons are living in close proximity, particularly if there is a regular supply of

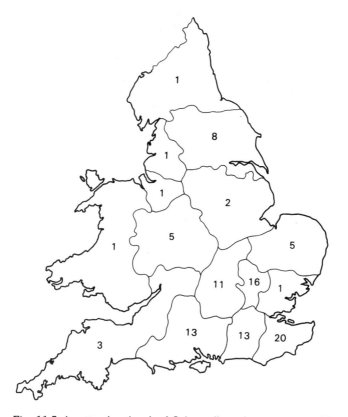

Fig. 11.5 A national outbreak of *Salmonella typhimurium* caused by contaminated salami sticks. Distribution of cases by NHS region (n = 101). (Source: Cowden J M, O'Mahoney M, Bartlett C L R *et al*. A national outbreak of *Salmonella typhimurium* caused by contaminated salami sticks. *Epidemiology of Infection* 1989; **103**: 219–225.

new susceptible individuals joining the community, e.g. nurseries, schools, military camps, etc. Different organisms and different strains of the same organism may vary in their virulence, the speed at which they spread, the carriage rate in a particular community and its duration in individuals.

Example
An example of the combined effect of these factors is the difference in epidemic behaviour exhibited by group B and group C strains of the meningococcus. Group B strains are characterized by low infectivity and slow transmission between susceptible hosts, low community carrier rates and high virulence. The result is that secondary cases within families and in communities such as schools, occur late and epidemics progress slowly and extend over long periods. For example, in an outbreak of group B type meningococcal disease in a primary school there were just four cases, two of them fatal over a 3-year period. Such associations, widely separated in time, may not be noticed until much damage has been done and very efficient systems of record keeping and registration are needed to avoid this. By contrast the group C meningococcus is characterized by rapid transmission and high carrier rates. In a closed community this may lead to large numbers of secondary cases in a relatively short time.

Remote communities tend to be relatively protected from some infections by their isolation. However, once infection is introduced it spreads with exceptional rapidity because herd immunity is usually low, e.g. respiratory infections in isolated island communities and Arctic expeditions which have been isolated for many months can cause very high morbidity rates. An epidemic may be initiated from a common source and then continue by secondary spread from person to person.

Example
An example of a propagated epidemic is an outbreak of measles that occurred in a primary school, shown in Fig. 11.6. Following two index cases in early

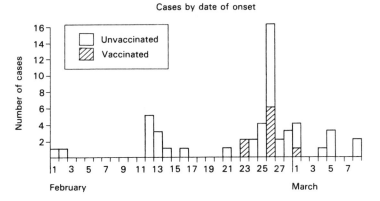

Fig. 11.6 Measles epidemic in a primary school. (From Graham R, Bellamy S, Richardson H J. *Communicable Disease Report* 1979; **16**)

February, there were two epidemic waves at approximately 10–14 day intervals, the median incubation period for measles. The outbreak was modified by the fact that many of the children in the school had been vaccinated, including some who contracted the disease. But the attack rate in unvaccinated children was high (86%) and showed the typical wave pattern of a propagated epidemic.

The investigation of outbreaks

Most epidemics are public health emergencies and require rapid and coordinated action to identify the cause and to institute effective control measures. It is wise to follow a systematic procedure in the investigation of outbreaks.

Outline of procedures

The steps described here are not necessarily undertaken in the sequence given. Enquiries usually proceed simultaneously with the analysis of findings and often with interim control measures based on early indications of the likely origin of the outbreak. Not all the steps will be relevant in every outbreak and the questions asked must be adapted to the circumstances. The four main stages in an investigation are:

descriptive enquiries into the facts of the outbreak;

analysis of the data collected;

formulation of a causal hypothesis;

testing its validity in the control of the outbreak.

Descriptive enquiries

- Verify the diagnosis by clinical and laboratory investigation of the cases.
- Verify the existence of an epidemic by comparison with previous incidence of the disease in the same population.
- Compile a list of all cases and search for unreported cases by alerting hospitals and general practitioners in the district and neighbouring districts.
- Investigate patients and others who might be involved in the outbreak. Record the personal characteristics of the patients (age, sex, address, etc) and enquire into shared experiences or activities that could carry risk of exposure to the suspected agent, e.g. occupation, school attended, recreational activities, consumption of foods, drugs, etc.
- Identify the total population at risk, that is all those who may have been exposed to the same hazards as the patients, whether ill or not.
- Ensure that all the clinical and laboratory investigations required to confirm the identity of the infection in patients and to determine the extent of sub-clinical infections are carried out. Phage and serological typing of organisms may help to establish the epidemiological association between cases and possible causes (or sources) and to trace the paths of spread of the agent.

Note

- The application of other epidemiological techniques such as the use of case-control studies may also be of value in the investigation of outbreaks as a means to confirm the validity of a causal hypothesis.

- In large outbreaks investigations can sometimes be confined to random samples of patients and persons thought to be at risk.

Investigate reservoirs and vehicles of infection which may be the source of the outbreak

Human

An epidemic may originate from an individual who has had a minor clinical episode or from a carrier who was ill many years previously. Therefore a careful history should be taken from *all* contacts of the patients.

Animal

Enquire about the contacts patients may have had with sick animals or animal products known to harbour the infection concerned.

Environment

Investigate sources of foods consumed by affected individuals and circumstances of their production, storage, preservation and preparation. Particular attention should be given to looking for situations in which cross-contamination or incubation of organisms could have occurred. Arrange for laboratory examination of food remnants, milk, and water supplies, and other relevant specimens from environmental sources, e.g. kitchen utensils, drains, etc, and the typing of any organisms that are isolated.

Analysis of the data collected

Plot of the epidemic curve

This may give some clue to the mode of spread and probable time of initial exposure.

Example

An outbreak of *Salmonella napoli* caused by contaminated chocolate bars imported from Italy is shown in Fig. 11.7. Note the relationship between the time distribution of cases and the importation of bars of chocolate.

Plot the cases on a map

This will detect clustering. The distribution of cases must be examined with reference to that of the population at risk.

Example

In an outbreak of legionellosis associated with an infected air conditioning plant on the roof of Broadcasting House in Central London the pattern of movement and hence possible points of exposure of cases were plotted on a grid map (Fig. 11.8). Broadcasting House, the suspected source of infection is in grid square C3. Note that the greatest density of places visited by the cases apart from C3 was in C4 and C5, which is a major shopping thoroughfare and in D2, D3 and D4 which are down wind from Broadcasting House.

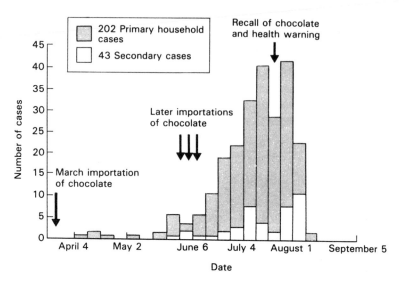

Fig. 11.7 Number of cases of infection with *Salmonella napoli* from chocolate during April–August 1982. (Source: Roberts J A, Sockett P N, Gill O N. Economic impact of a nationwide outbreak of salmonellosis: cost–benefit of early intervention. *Br Med J 1989;* **289**: 1227.)

Analyse the incidence rates in different groups

This can be done, for example, for age or occupation. A high rate in a particular group suggests that the cause lies in a common experience of its members. Attack rates must be calculated both in those exposed and in those not exposed to the suspected agent. It should be noted that variations in the biological response may result in attack rates of less than 100% in the exposed population.

Look for a quantitative relationship

This may exist between the degree of exposure (or dose) and attack rate, e.g. amount of suspect food consumed or closeness to a source of pollution.

Example

In an outbreak of foodborne viral gastroenteritis, food histories were obtained from 239 guests at the suspect meal. Of these guests, 206 reported illness. The food-specific attack rates showed clearly that the melon was the probable vehicle of infection (Table 11.1).

Formulation of a causal hypothesis

The hypothesis should take account of:
• The properties of the agent, its reservoirs and favoured vehicles and also of the nature of the illness it causes.
• The probable route of transmission, in this instance the typing of the organisms may be particularly helpful.

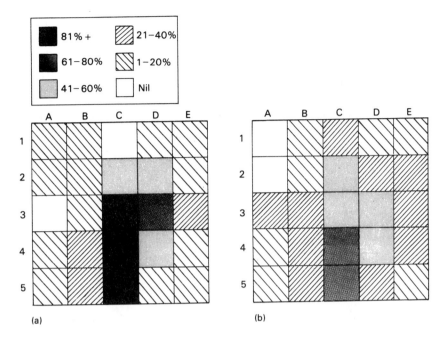

Fig. 11.8 Proportions of people giving definite answers who had visited grid areas in the 10 days before onset of illness. (a) BBC staff and contractors. All pneumonias and legionella illness (36). (b) Non-BBC. Confirmed cases of legionnaires disease only (46). (Source: Report of the Westminster Action Committee convened to co-ordinate the investigation and control of the outbreak of legionnaires disease associated with Portland Place, London W1 in April–May 1988.)

Table 11.1 Outbreak of viral foodborne gastroenteritis: food-specific attack rates. (Source: Iverson A M, Gill M, Bartlett C L R, Cubitt W D, McSwiggan D. Two outbreaks of foodborne gastroenteritis by a small round structured virus: evidence of prolonged infectivity in a food handler. *Lancet* **ii**: 556.)

Food*	Ate		Did not eat		p value[†]
	Ill	Not ill	Ill	Not ill	
Melon	197	23	0	5	0.000006
Beef	196	27	4	1	NS
Potatoes	196	22	3	6	NS
Horseradish sauce	142	19	58	9	NS
Blackforest gâteau	184	23	16	5	NS
Cream	180	22	19	7	NS

*Main items only—none of the original foods were associated with illness.
[†]Fishers exact test. NS = not significant.

- Time and duration of exposure of the patients to the agent in relation to the onset of their illness.
- Attack rates of the different sub-group of the population at risk

Testing validity in the control of the outbreak

Seek support for the hypothesis by further investigation of cases, if necessary, to confirm the proposed explanation of their illness. Carefully designed case-control studies may be very helpful in this.

Implement appropriate control measures on the assumption that the hypothesis is correct and monitor their success in reducing the incidence of further cases.

Chapter 12
Occupational Health and Accidents

OCCUPATIONAL HEALTH

Introduction

More than half the population of Britain spends at least 38 hours a week at work outside their homes. Consequently the safety of the working environment and its possible adverse effects on health are matters of great significance. However, despite much genuine public concern for safety at work and the existence of extensive legislation aimed at protecting workers, the attention given to the health of workers and the standards of safety that are applied vary widely.

In some diseases, attributable to the victim's occupation, the causes are known and specific and their effects are rapidly apparent. However, most occupational diseases tend to be the result of chronic exposures with long latent periods. In these circumstances, it can be difficult or impossible to differentiate between the occupational exposure and other exposures unrelated to the workplace. For example, bronchitis amongst steel workers who also smoke. Even when a specific hazard is known and the method of prevention is clear, its application and consequently its effectiveness often depends on persuading employers and employees to act in ways which may reduce profitability or earning capacity. Legislation may help, but changing human behaviour in ways that people are disinclined to follow is a critical element in prevention.

Occupational hazards

The range of potential hazards associated with different occupations is enormous and is not dealt with here in any detail. There are some specific dangers such as those related to handling, ingestion or inhalation of noxious substances, e.g. dusts, fumes, poisons and pathogenic organisms, radiation, excessive noise and accidents with machinery which can be identified easily. Such physical hazards are usually simple to prevent. Others, e.g. chemical carcinogens with a long latent interval, (such as the association of nasal cancer with the occupation of furniture making), require careful epidemiological study for their recognition.

It is considerably more difficult to define and deal with numerous other environmental conditions affecting health and efficiency in subtle ways, often more through psychological than physical damage. For example, uncomfortably hot or cold surroundings, poor lighting, noisy machinery, repetitive and uninteresting tasks, and excessive fatigue, all tend to be associated with increased accident rates, sickness absence and staff turnover, as well as with reduced productivity. Mental health also is affected by such factors as job satisfaction, boredom, degree of isolation and stressful relationships with colleagues.

Principles of prevention of ill health related to occupation

Primary responsibility for safe working conditions rests with the employer; preventive action which depends on the worker tends to be less successful. There are three possible strategies:

1 substitute safe for harmful working conditions;
2 protect workers from the effects of dangers in their environment;
3 monitor the concentration of known harmful agents in the working environment and, where applicable, in the tissues of workers;

Screening for early detection for disease (see p. 155) may be necessary where the other strategies are not practicable or cannot be totally relied on to avert the risk that some workers will develop disease.

Substitution

Where there is a clearly harmful material or process, it should if possible, be replaced by a safe one. For example, asbestos is now being replaced by other insulating materials and shot-blasting is replacing sand-blasting in order to prevent silicosis.

Protection

If the agent cannot be completely removed, then the workers should be protected from its dangers. There are several ways of doing this:

Enclosure

Dangerous processes or machinery can be enclosed. For example, processes which involve the use of radioactive substances, toxic chemicals or the production of harmful fumes should be conducted in effectively sealed containers. Similarly moving parts of machinery should be adequately guarded.

Segregation

If total enclosure is not possible, hazardous processes should be carried out in segregated locations. For example, dangerous pathogens such as rabies, lassa fever and Marburg viruses should be handled only in laboratories with effective security. In this way the numbers of workers at risk can be restricted to those who are trained in safe practices. In some cases the duration of exposure of individual workers to harmful agents is limited for their own protection, e.g. where a risk of significant radiation is involved.

Ventilation

Where the isolation of processes is impracticable exposure to toxic fumes and dusts are reduced by efficient exhaust ventilation. Ventilation also reduces the concentration of noxious gases by dilution and thereby reduces the risk of their causing harm.

Lighting and temperature

Good lighting and comfortable working temperatures help to reduce accidents and stress on workers.

Shielding the worker

It is often not practical to devise totally safe processes and, in this case, it is necessary to shield the worker, e.g. by the use of protective clothing, respirators, goggles, helmets, ear plugs or barrier creams. Unfortunately, such equipment is often hot and uncomfortable to wear, it restricts movement and sometimes vision, and it slows workers down, thereby tending to reduce their earning capacity, which discourages its use.

Cleanliness and tidiness

Cleanliness and tidiness in workshops reduces both the chances of exposure to dangerous substances and the risk of accidents. Similarly, attention to hygiene, washing hands or showering, if indicated, avoidance of smoking and eating in workplaces are important preventive measures in many situations.

General working conditions

General working conditions may also be almost as important in the prevention of ill health attributable to occupation as physical dangers. Attention should therefore be given to such matters as comfort and pleasantness of the environment, e.g. in offices, interest of tasks, e.g. on production lines, limitation of hours of work to avoid excessive fatigue, e.g. for transport drivers, and companionship at work.

Monitoring

In order to reduce the risks of harm to workers by exposure to particular toxic substances, careful monitoring should be practised. This may be either by measurement of the concentration of toxic substances in the environment or by biological observations in workers.

Environmental monitoring

Environmental monitoring is applied mainly to airborne substances. The assumption is made that if environmental concentrations are maintained below a certain level the risk of harm to exposed workers will be negligible. For this purpose two sets of values have been established for a wide range of toxic substances:

- *Threshold limit values*

These are maximum time-weighted average concentrations to which a worker may be exposed during a normal working day. Because of biological variation, a threshold limit value (TLV) cannot ensure safety in all workers, and it is prudent to keep as far below the TLV as is practical.

- *Ceiling values*

These are concentrations which must not be exceeded at any time.

It should be realized that both indices may be exceeded in local situations which might not be detected by general environmental monitoring. Where this possibility exists workers should wear personal monitors to measure their individual exposure, e.g. workers exposed to radiation risks.

Biological monitoring

This is concerned with measurement of the amounts of a toxic substance actually absorbed by the body or the early detection of an adverse effect induced by occupational exposure. Examples of this are the estimation of blood lead concentrations in workers engaged in processes connected with lead; audiometry in those exposed to high noise intensity; proteinuria for tubular function in cadmium workers. The Employment Medical Advisory Service issues lists of suggested *biological threshold values* for certain substances, but the degree of deviation from normal values which can be tolerated before damage occurs is often disputed and probably varies between individuals.

Occupational health services

Although employers are not required to provide occupational health services they exist in many large organizations. Sometimes the service is staffed by doctors; otherwise it is provided by nurses with part-time help from local general practitioners. There are a few group industrial health services which provide small firms with services on a contract basis.

Occupational health services usually provide emergency services for workers who are taken ill or suffer accidents at work, and also provide preventive advice to management and workers. Another function is the conduct of pre-employment and routine medical examinations for certain categories of workers who are exposed to special hazards, some of which are required by law. The value of pre-employment medical examinations is controversial. The main aims are to assess an individual's fitness to undertake the work he will do and to provide base-line observations against which to compare the results of future examinations. Some medical examinations are designed to protect the public as much as the worker, e.g. the examination of faecal samples in water supply workers and food handlers, and the stringent medical examinations required for air crew.

Legislation and occupational health

Legislation governing working conditions has been voluminous and complex, having been built up piecemeal since the industrial revolution. It covers such topics as space, ventilation, lighting, heating and cleanliness in work places, guards on machinery, safety appliances, fire regulations, the provision of sanitary and washing accommodation and of first aid facilities, and the medical examination and biological monitoring of workers in certain occupations. Responsibility for supervising the implementation of much of this legislation rested in the past with seven inspectorates set up under various government departments. Of these the Factory Inspectorate, established in 1833, was the oldest and largest. The old, cumbersome legislation was replaced by the Health and Safety at Work Act (1974), a comprehensive, enabling Act giving wide powers which apply to all work places. It affects both employees and employers, includes responsibility for the protection of the general environment from the effects of industrial processes, and requires employers to notify accidents. The work of the Inspectorates, including the Employment Medical Advisory Service, is now enforced under the Health and Safety Commission set up under the Act.

Employment Medical Advisory Service

This service was formed from the medical branch of the Factory Inspectorate in 1973. Its functions are to advise employers, employees, unions and doctors on all medical problems related to work. It is responsible for ensuring that periodic medical examinations are carried out on workers in certain hazardous processes, e.g. lead workers, and on any employee whose health is believed to be in danger because of his work. The service is also responsible for advising school leavers with health problems on choice of employment, advising on disablement resettlement services and providing medical supervision at industrial rehabilitation units.

ACCIDENTS

Introduction

In England and Wales accidents result in about 22 000 deaths, 500 000 hospital admissions and 27 million days lost from work each year. There is substantial variation in the numbers and in the types of accident with age and sex. This is exemplified by the mortality statistics shown in Table 12.1.

The pattern of accidents varies enormously with environmental conditions and personal factors. For example, road accidents occur most frequently in the hours of darkness and in winter months, whereas drownings occur most frequently in the daytime in summer. Nearly half of all deaths in children are the result of traffic accidents, except in those under 5 years old in whom suffocation is the most common cause, followed by burns and scalds, falls and poisoning. There is a sharp peak in the incidence of road accident deaths in males in the 15–24 year age group, due in particular to motor cycle accidents. This peak is much less dramatic in females. In persons over 65, the frequency of accidental

Table 12.1 Deaths from accidents in England and Wales (1986). Numbers and percentages by place of accident

	Age (years)							
	Males				Females			
	0–14	15–44	45–64	65 +	0–14	15–44	45–64	65 +
Numbers	462	3575	1425	2120	261	1017	729	3376
Percentages								
Road	51.3	57.4	37.1	28.7	51.7	51.3	30.9	17.2
Home and residential	30.1	18.1	30.7	48.5	34.9	30.1	45.5	61.1
Industrial	0.6	4.4	6.7	0.7	0.8	0.5	0.5	0.3
Public places	5.0	4.7	5.5	4.8	5.4	2.6	2.9	2.7
Other	13.0	15.4	20.1	17.4	7.3	15.5	20.2	18.7

deaths increases, particularly as a result of falls in females. Statistics such as these help to identify areas of risk in which there is a special need for preventive effort.

The prevention of accidents rests first on the provision of a safe environment, second, on the education of people in safe practices, and third, on regulation of environmental conditions and of the behaviour of individuals by legal sanctions.

Environmental safety

It is always preferable to create a safe environment than to rely on public education in safety. This is exemplified by action taken to improve road and home safety.

Road safety

This has been enhanced by improvements in road engineering, surfaces and furnishings, better street lighting, combined with safety devices in the design of vehicles.

Home safety

This has been improved by better design of domestic appliances (especially electrical and heating appliances), flame-proof children's clothing, good housing design (especially the protection of stairs and balconies). Prevention also depends on maintaining the home and its contents in a good state of repair, e.g. electrical wiring, lighting and carpets, especially on stairs.

Education

While the safety of the environment is of paramount importance, not all dangers can be removed. Therefore, individuals must be taught the nature of dangers in the environment and how to reduce them. Educational programmes on safety feature increasingly in schools, the media and in the activities of health education units. For example:

Road safety

The Green Cross Code for children and the Highway Code for adult road users offer guidance in the safe use of roads.

Home safety

Building regulations govern their safety in relation to fire hazards, ventilation, lighting and other matters. Regulations on the safety of domestic appliances also indirectly assist safety in the home.

Mothers should be taught the dangers to children from inhalable objects and plastic bags, the need for guards on all fires, care in keeping drugs and chemical cleaning compounds in 'child-proof' containers and out of their reach. The elderly are particularly susceptible to accidents by reason of defective hearing, vision, physical infirmity and forgetfulness and need to be encouraged in safe habits. These are important aspects of the role which health visitors and general practitioners can play during visits to households with small children and elderly people.

It should be noted that environmental control, education and regulation are insufficient to eliminate accidents in certain circumstances. For example, many motor cycle accidents are caused not by people using the motor cycle as a method of transport but as a way of testing nerve during late adolescence, almost amounting to a cult. Those who pursue these dangerous activities are well aware of the risks, and are prepared to accept the personal risks involved in exactly the same way as a mountaineer. Nor do they regard the risks imposed on others as a significant deterrent. The desire of adolescents to test the limits of their physical endurance is a natural phenomenon and hard to combat by any conventional preventive strategies.

Regulation

There is much value in the legal regulation of environmental conditions and some dangerous aspects of public behaviour. For example:

Road safety

The 1967 Road Safety Act introduced regulations relating to drinking and driving. This was followed by a substantial fall in the number of serious accidents. Many countries have introduced laws making the wearing of seat belts compulsory for car drivers and front seat passengers with the result that deaths and serious injuries from road accidents have been significantly reduced. Legislation already exists in Britain relating to worn tyres and other vehicle safety features; motor cyclists are required to wear crash helmets. Enforcement of these regulations, however, presents serious practical difficulties and their effectiveness is therefore limited.

Chapter 13
Immunization

Introduction

The resistance of susceptible individuals to certain bacterial and viral infections can be artificially enhanced either by passive or by active immunization.

Passive immunization

This is the donation to the host of specific antibodies against a particular agent by the injection of blood products derived from immune animals or humans. It is used to give a degree of immediate, though temporary, protection to non-immune patients who have been recently exposed to a potentially dangerous infection. Active immunization is not appropriate in these circumstances because of the lag period between the administration of vaccine and the production of antibodies in protective amounts.

Products used for passive immunization are immunoglobulins which are now normally derived from the blood of human donors. The practice of using animal (usually horse) sera for this purpose has generally been abandoned because of the risk of anaphylaxis. The degree and duration of the protection afforded depends on the amount of antibody present, but significant protection usually lasts no more than 3–6 months. Human normal immunoglobulin (HNIG) is extracted from pooled plasma from blood donors. It contains antibodies active against measles, mumps, varicella, hepatitis and other viruses commonly occurring in the general population. Specific immunoglobulins active against varicella, tetanus, rabies or hepatitis B are prepared from the pooled blood of individuals who have recently suffered an attack of, or have been actively immunized against the particular disease. All these products are expensive and in short supply. Their use must, therefore, be carefully controlled.

Active immunization

This involves the administration of appropriate vaccines which stimulate the production by the host of specific protective antibodies. This provides complete or partial protection, usually lasting at least for a few years and in some cases for life. Active immunization is usually given as a planned procedure. It is designed both to protect individuals against infections to which they may be exposed at some time in the future and to control the spread of infection in the community.

The production of antibodies after the first dose of some types of vaccine tends to be slow and inadequate. Multiple doses at intervals of days or weeks are required to achieve protective levels of antibody. Further reinforcing doses at intervals may be necessary to maintain immunity. Such doses (or later natural infection) stimulate an antibody response which is always more rapid and usually greater and more durable than the primary response.

Vaccines

Vaccines are of three main types:
inactivated vaccines;
live vaccines;
toxoids.

Inactivated vaccines

These are made from organisms killed during manufacture. Examples include pertussis, injected (Salk) poliomyelitis, typhoid and cholera vaccines.

Live vaccines

These are made from living organisms which are either:
- Organisms which cause the disease whose virulence has been reduced by attenuation. Examples include oral (Sabin) poliomyelitis, measles and rubella vaccines.
- Organisms of a species antigenically related to the causal agent but which are naturally less virulent. Examples: smallpox (vaccinia) and tuberculosis (BCG) vaccines.

Toxoids

These are produced from bacterial toxins artificially rendered harmless. Examples include diphtheria and tetanus vaccines.

Vaccines vary in their antigenic potency, that is their capacity to induce the formation of protective antibody. This can sometimes be enhanced by adjuvants such as aluminium phosphate and aluminium hydroxide which are used with the diphtheria, tetanus, pertussis (DTP), or 'Triple' vaccine.

The route of administration varies between vaccines, most are injected into or under the skin. Live polio vaccine is given orally which has the advantage of stimulating local immunity in the intestine which inhibits later colonization (and transmission) of wild polio virus.

In order to reduce the number of separate injections several agents are sometimes incorporated in the same vaccine, for example DTP vaccine which includes pertussis vaccine with tetanus and diphtheria toxoids and MMR which includes measles, mumps and rubella vaccines. It is sometimes thought to be unwise to give two live vaccines together because of a possible increased risk of adverse reactions. Therefore, when giving more than one such vaccine it is still considered advisable either to give them simultaneously in different sites (unless a combined preparation is used) or to separate them by an interval of not less than 3 weeks.

Routine immunization

The schedule for routine immunization recommended in the UK is shown in Table 13.1. The exact timing of doses is open to variation. While the ages recommended for each vaccine are considered to be optimum, it is important to ensure as far as possible that all children are vaccinated even if they present

Table 13.1 Schedule of routine childhood immunization in the UK. (For further details *see Immunisation Against Infectious Disease*. Department of Health, Welsh and Scottish Home and Health Department, HMSO, London, 1990.)

Vaccine	Age	Notes
Diphtheria/tetanus/pertussis (DTP or 'triple') and oral polio (OPV)		
Dose 1 Dose 2 Dose 3	2 months 3 months 4 months	*All* children should be vaccinated (in absence of specific contraindications) with full primary course even if younger or older than recommended age-range
Measles/mumps/rubella (MMR)	12–18 months	Can be given at any age over 12 months
Booster diptheria/tetanus and polio	4–5 years (School entry)	
Rubella	10–14 years	*Girls only*
BCG	10–14 years Infants at high risk	Interval of 3 weeks between BCG and rubella vaccine
Booster tetanus and polio	15–18 years	

outside the recommended age range, unless there are specific contraindications (see *Immunisation Against Infectious Disease,* HMSO 1990).

Diphtheria, tetanus, pertussis, and poliomyelitis

In order to ensure protection against these diseases as early in infancy as possible, especially whooping cough which is most serious in the first months of life, it is now considered that primary immunization with DTP and oral polio vaccine should begin at the age of 2 months and be completed by 4 months. Previous fears about the safety of pertussis vaccine are now largely discounted and any possible risk attached to the vaccine is considered to be slight in relation to the risks of the disease.

Reinforcing doses of diphtheria/tetanus (DT) and oral polio vaccine (OPV) should be given at or shortly before school entry. Further doses of tetanus and OPV are required at 15–18 years. Further reinforcing doses of tetanus vaccine may be required after certain types of high risk injury or burns occurring in individuals immunized more than 5 years previously. Where an individual with such an injury has no clear history of having completed a primary course of tetanus immunization a dose of human anti-tetanus immunoglobulin should be given at the same time as the first dose of a primary course of active immunization.

Adults who have not been immunized against poliomyelitis in childhood should receive a primary course of three doses of OPV: no adult should be left unprotected against polio. Further reinforcing doses after that given at 15–18 years are not normally required, exceptions are travellers to countries where the disease is epidemic or endemic and health care workers in possible contact with cases of the disease.

Measles, mumps and rubella vaccine (MMR)

Measles is an acute viral illness which is highly infectious in unvaccinated children. It is a major cause of childhood morbidity which, in the period 1970–1980 caused an average of 13 deaths a year in England and Wales. Complications occur in 1 in 15 reported cases and include encephalitis, otitis media, pneumonia and bronchitis. Measles is thus, potentially, a major cause of acute and chronic ill health in children. Measles vaccine was introduced to the UK in 1968. It is administered shortly after the first birthday. Earlier administration is not advised because of the presence of maternal antibody.

Maternal rubella infection in the first 8–10 weeks of pregnancy results in fetal damage in up to 90% of infants and multiple defects are common. The risk of damage declines to about 10–20% by 16 weeks gestation after which fetal damage is rare. Rubella vaccine was introduced in the UK in 1970 and has since been recommended for all girls aged between 10 and 14 years of age and for non-pregnant sero-negative women of child bearing age. The application of this policy over the years since 1970 had increased the proportion of ante-natal women with the rubella antibody to 97–98% by 1987. Amongst the remaining 2% however, 362 cases of rubella infection in pregnancy were recorded in 1986 and 1987 in England and Wales. Many of these pregnancies were terminated but on average 20 cases of congenital rubella syndrome (CRS) are still notified annually. Thus, the original policy of selective vaccination for girls and women has been only partially successful. This policy was intended to protect women of child bearing age while permitting the continued circulation of wild rubella virus in the community in order to provide continued stimulation of the immune system of vaccinated females and boost the original vaccine-induce immunity. From 1988 when MMR vaccine was introduced, both boys and girls are being offered vaccination against measles, mumps and rubella in early childhood. The aim is to *eliminate* measles, mumps, rubella and CRS. The policy of vaccinating girls between the age of 10 and 14 years and non-immune non-pregnant women will continue for the time being. When a high uptake, i.e. 90% or more, of MMR vaccine in children has been achieved and maintained and the elimination of rubella has been demonstrated it may be reasonable to stop the vaccination of schoolgirls.

Tuberculosis: BCG vaccine

BCG vaccine is recommended for *tuberculin negative* persons in the following categories:
- Contacts of cases known to be suffering from active respiratory tuberculosis. The children of immigrants in whose communities there is a high incidence of

tuberculosis may for this purpose be regarded as contacts. Newborn babies who are contacts, need not be tested for tuberculin sensitivity but should be vaccinated without delay.

• Health service staff: this category should include medical students, hospital medical staff, nurses, and any other staff who come into contact with patients (physiotherapists, radiographers, technical staff in pathology departments). It is particularly important to test staff working in maternity and paediatric departments.

Other non-routine vaccines

Anthrax

This is an effective vaccine recommended only for workers at occupational risk of exposure to infection. They should also use protective clothing and environmental measures to control dust. Adequate ventilation should be provided.

Cholera

This vaccine is made from killed organisms and is required for travel to certain countries where cholera occurs. Immunity is short-lived and immunizations should be repeated every 6 months where exposure continues.

Hepatitis B

This vaccine is about 90% effective overall; it is slightly less effective in those over 40 years of age than in younger people. The duration of vaccine-induced immunity is thought to be 3–5 years. It is recommended for doctors, dentists, nurses, midwives and other health service staff including students and porters who have direct contact with patients or their body fluids or who are likely to experience exposure to blood or blood contaminated secretions and excretions. It is also advisable for patients on entry to units dealing with the mentally handicapped, laboratory workers and mortuary technicians, renal dialysis patients, the sexual partners of hepatitis B carriers and infants whose mothers are carriers. Parenteral drug abusers, prostitutes and other sexually promiscuous individuals of both sexes, morticians and embalmers, inmates of long-term custodial institutions, travellers to areas of the world where the disease is endemic and certain members of the police and other emergency services judged to be at high risk may also be considered for vaccination.

Influenza

Evidence of the protective value of influenza vaccines is conflicting. Vaccine prepared from the latest antigenic variants of influenza A and B virus is recommended in the early autumn for persons at special risk, such as the elderly (especially those living in residential institutions) and for those suffering from certain chronic diseases including pulmonary, cardiac and renal disease, diabetes and other endocrine disorders and conditions requiring immunosuppressive therapy. The vaccine is not recommended for the control of outbreaks. Live influenza vaccines are still regarded as experimental and are not in general use in this country.

Rabies

This is usually given combined with passive immunization with rabies immuno-globulin only to persons bitten by a rabid animal or by one thought to be infected. It may also be offered to those with a high occupational risk.

Smallpox

With the success of the WHO smallpox eradication programme the use of the vaccine is no longer recommended.

Typhoid

Monovalent typhoid vaccine given by intramuscular or deep subcutaneous injection provides 70–80% protection which fades after 1 year. A second dose given 4–6 weeks later provides protection for 3 or more years. The vaccine is recommended for laboratory workers handling specimens which contain the organism and for persons travelling to countries of high risk. Under conditions of continued or repeated exposure to infection a reinforcing dose should be given every 3 years.

Yellow fever

This vaccine contains a live attenuated virus. It is indicated only for those people visiting yellow fever infected areas, i.e. parts of Central and South America and Equatorial Africa. Laboratory workers handling infected material should also be vaccinated.

Additional note on protection for travellers

A reinforcing dose of polio vaccine is advisable before travel to some tropical countries. Consideration should also be given to the need for immunoglobulin to protect against infectious hepatitis and for malaria prophylaxis where appropriate.

Safety and efficacy of vaccines

Although no new vaccine is released without extensive safety tests in animals and controlled field trials, there remains some risk of adverse reactions. Careful observance of specific contraindications to each particular vaccine reduces the risk. Nevertheless, some vaccines not infrequently give rise to minor reactions, e.g. local oedema at the injection site, transient fever or rash. The very rare neurological conditions that may arise after almost any vaccine are of greater concern. To assess their significance routine surveillance must be maintained. Careful records should be kept of all the vaccinations given, to whom and where, with particulars of the vaccine used, and any serious reactions should be reported at once to the Committee on Safety of Medicines. Likewise the continued efficacy of a vaccine in controlling a disease should be monitored by the analysis of routine morbidity and mortality reports and, where appropriate, by microbiological and antibody surveys. This is undertaken at the CDSC of the PHLS in London.

Vaccination targets

In *Health for all by the year 2000*, WHO states its aim that indigenous poliomyelitis, measles, neonatal tetanus, CRS and diphtheria should have been eradicated from the European region by that date. To achieve this UK Health Departments have set as their target that 95% of the child population will be immunized against the common infectious diseases by that date. Vaccination programmes tend to be less successful in the lower socio-economic and mobile groups, resulting in pockets of susceptible individuals amongst whom the spread of infection can persist. They also tend to be difficult to sustain in communities which have little or no recent experience of the disease in question. In such communities the problems of safety tend to loom larger in the public consciousness than the problems of the disease. Professional attitudes and motivation also influence uptake rates. The uptake of vaccination against measles and whooping cough in the UK was until recently comparatively low. One cause of this poor performance was the prevalence of false information and myths about contraindications among responsible professionals. In the USA a system has been adopted whereby evidence of having completed the recommended vaccination and immunization programme is required before a child is allowed to enter school. As a result very high immunization rates in the child population have been achieved leading to the virtual eradication of the preventable diseases of childhood. Compulsion of this kind is thought by many to be alien to the British tradition and to propose its introduction would certainly arouse controversy. Nevertheless, parents who refuse vaccination for their children should be aware that not only do they put their own children at risk but also help to perpetuate a hazard to the community as a whole.

Chapter 14
Health Education and Nutrition

HEALTH EDUCATION AND HEALTH PROMOTION

Introduction

Health education attempts to influence the attitudes and behaviour of individuals and of communities by increasing their knowledge and understanding of health and diseases. It is important because prevention of many diseases and the promotion of positive health can only be effected by a combination of the personal commitment of individuals and the informed consent of the community backed where necessary by appropriate governmental action. Health education and legal direction was recognized as being of great value in ancient civilizations: much Hebrew Law for example incorporates useful public health teaching, e.g. Leviticus, Chapter 11.

The specific objectives of health education are as follows.

- To increase knowledge of the factors that affect health.
- To encourage behaviour which promotes and maintains health.
- To enlist support for public health measures and, where necessary, to press for appropriate government action.
- To educate people to recognize the early signs of disease and to take remedial action.
- To encourage appropriate use of health services especially preventative services.
- To inform the public about medical advances, their uses and their limitations.

These objectives are often frustrated by public suspicion of those who would 'do them good' and reflex resistance to any interference with personal freedom. To the public there seems to be an ever lengthening list of deprecated habits, e.g. smoking, drinking, eating to excess, and sloth, many of which are pleasurable. Health education must always be tempered by sensitivity to the right of individuals to free choice in matters of behaviour, provided it is not likely to be harmful to other people or to the interests of society as a whole. Success will depend heavily on an understanding of what motivates people to change their behaviour. It is also sometimes necessary to persuade people to subject themselves to screening or pre-emptive therapy at time when they believe themselves to be fit.

A further difficulty is that convincing evidence for the beneficial effects of changing existing patterns of life is often lacking and medical opinion often appears to be divided and prone to periodic changes. Therefore, it is important to stress the positive advantages of restricting harmful habits and to concentrate on diseases in which there is most to be gained by modification of behaviour.

Health education programmes

There are some specific programmes that are generally accepted as being of value. Examples of these are listed below.

Health promotion

The instruction of expectant mothers in the physiology of pregnancy and parturition during their attendance at antenatal clinics enhances their confidence and leads to a more relaxed confinement.

The health visitor system has improved child rearing practices. In earlier times such 'education' as this was given informally within the extended family but in modern urban society the 'family' is often insufficiently preserved to be effective in this respect.

Keep fit classes and other leisure activity programmes have made many people more aware of the benefits of a more positive approach to health.

Pre-retirement courses are useful in preparation for old age.

The prevention and alleviation of specific diseases

The association between cigarette smoking and lung cancer, cardiovascular disease and some other conditions has been amply demonstrated and campaigns aimed at persuading people to stop smoking have shown benefits.

The control of food poisoning owes much to improved public understanding of how these diseases are transmitted, leading to improved standards of hygiene in the home as well as in the food industry.

The incidence of alcoholism and related diseases has increased greatly in recent years and persuading people to moderate their intake of alcohol is likely to be one of the major tasks of health education in future.

Persuasion of the public to accept legislation

Without the strict laws which govern the sale and consumption of drugs the problems of addiction would be immensely greater. Although it is hard to dissuade many people from drinking and driving, public opinion was prepared to accept legislation against this potentially dangerous practice.

Health educationalists are active in persuading people and water authorities to accept fluoridation of water supplies as a means of reducing dental caries.

Encouragement in the efficient use of health services

Health services are not always used appropriately. For example, Accident and Emergency Services are frequently used by patients for complaints that could be better dealt with by their general practitioner. Similarly, some of those in need of health services are unfamiliar with the relevant care systems, for example ethnic minority groups. Immunization and certain screening programmes for presymptomatic disease are good examples of preventive services whose success depends on high acceptance rates. This requires a continuing major educational effort.

Methods of health education

To succeed in health education it is essential to have:

- Insight into the social and psychological determinants of human behaviour.
- A clear message. This means deciding at the outset what information is to be communicated and what change in behaviour is desired.
- Good communication technique. The facts given should be truthful, accurate and clearly distinguished from opinion. The presentation must be simple and devoid of technical jargon.

Health education can be provided either on an individual basis, to groups of people, or to the population as a whole (mass education).

Individual education

Doctors (particularly general practitioners) nurses and health visitors have daily opportunities to instruct patients and answer their questions during the course of normal care. Such direct approaches from respected authorities, who often have close personal relationships with patients, are probably the most influential. They have the particular advantage that sick individuals are actively seeking information and advice about prevention and therefore are likely to be more receptive than those at present in good health. The example of health professionals in such matters as smoking is perhaps particularly important.

Group health education

Some organized health education is conducted in groups, e.g. in schools, child health clinics and industry. School teachers, health visitors, social workers and industrial medical officers are experienced in the art of communication and there is much to be said for health education being included in the course of other education and training activities.

Mass education

The power of advertising through the mass media in shaping attitudes is indisputable. The prohibition or restriction of advertising which encourages harmful activities is as important as using the media for health education, but the budget available to commerce far exceeds that available to health educationalists. Health documentaries and drama relating to medicine have a continuing public appeal which can be harnessed to the advantage of health education.

Organization of health education

Statutory

Health authorities are responsible for providing a health education service within their districts. Local education authorities are responsible for the inclusion of the subject in school curricula.

The Health Education Authority

This is a special health authority of the NHS in England, having taken over the responsibilities of the former Health Education Council on 1st April 1987. From October 1987 it assumed responsibility for public health education on AIDS.

The Authority leads and supports promotion of health in England. The aims are:

- to increase the knowledge and understanding in society of the factors which contribute to health and disease, and how health might be promoted and disease reduced;
- to influence individuals and organizations to take whatever action lies within their power to improve health and reduce disease.

The main functions are:

- to advise the Secretary of State for Health on matters related to health education;
- to undertake health education activities;
- for the purpose of planning and carrying out national and regional or local programmes or other activities in cooperation with health authorities, voluntary organizations and other persons or bodies concerned with health education;
- to assist in the provision of appropriate training in health education;
- to prepare, publish, and distribute material relevant to health education;
- to provide a national centre of information and advice on health education.

Members of the Board of the Authority are appointed by the Secretary of State for Health for a period not exceeding 4 years. They include leading figures from health associated professions, the media, education and other related fields.

Voluntary bodies

A number of voluntary bodies, such as the Royal Society for the Prevention of Accidents, are concerned with specific aspects of public education in matters of health.

NUTRITIONAL POLICY AND ADVICE

Although the relationship between diet and health is complex the importance of good nutrition in the prevention of disease and in the promotion of health is beyond doubt.

Malnutrition

Chronic malnutrition was commonplace in Britain before the industrial revolution. As in all developed countries it is now rare. There are, however, large parts of the world where supplies of basic foods are seriously inadequate and where famine and death from starvation still occur. In some countries where food supplies only just keep pace with demand, natural disasters such as flood, earthquakes or drought, can precipitate grave problems of malnutrition. The continued increase in world population will further increase demands on food supplies and unless radical steps are taken, the situation will worsen. Poverty, whether national or personal, limits not only the quantity of food but also reduces the choice and quality. In such circumstances people tend to eat what food they can get without paying too much attention to its nutritional content. The results may be an unbalanced diet containing an excessive proportion of cheap carbohydrates and seriously deficient in essential constituents such as proteins and vitamins. Even when supplies of food are adequate, dietary composition is influenced by culture and by tradition. There are many examples of strong religious taboos in relation to diet and most communities develop their local customs and tastes in food.

Individual needs

The quantity of food and the amounts of different constituents that are required for health vary between individuals. Obviously the needs of babies, infants, children, active adults and the elderly differ and people involved in strenuous physical activity will require more energy-producing foods. Where there is a plentiful supply, adjustments in relation to needs are made without conscious effort, but in famine situations children can be irreparably damaged in a relatively short period of time. They are always the most vulnerable members of the population in times of hardship. Women also require relatively more food and greater amounts of certain constituents, e.g. iron, when pregnant than at other times; their dietary balance is of great importance because of its potential effect on the unborn child. Where there is extreme dietary deficiency people are more susceptible to infection and the consequences of infection are more serious. For example, measles is more severe and more often fatal in malnourished children.

Children in Britain

In Britain, the problem of malnutrition in children at the beginning of the century was highlighted when it was found that about half of army recruits at the time of the Boer War were rejected on medical grounds. This finding led to the establishment of a school meals service which was free to the children of poor families. Attention to the quality of diet was later stimulated by evidence of the enhanced growth of children who were given extra milk. These benefits together with the provision of cheap milk and welfare foods for expectant and nursing mothers and pre-school children contributed to the improvement in health of the child population, particularly the poor. However, such dietary supplements are now considered to be unnecessary for children taking an average normal diet in Britain today.

The elderly

Another group that is especially vulnerable to malnutrition is the elderly, particularly those who live alone. This is partly because of poverty among them; it is also because of their disabilities, immobility, lack of cooking facilities and indifference to food. To meet their needs, cooked meals (free or at a modest charge) were provided by the Women's Royal Voluntary Service 'Meals on Wheels' service and through luncheon clubs for both of which local authority social services departments are now responsible.

Excess in eating

Evidence has accumulated in recent years on the dangers to health of excessive eating. Those who are overweight suffer from an increased incidence of mechanical disorders, such as arthritis, varicose veins and the effects of impaired mobility. Obesity is also associated with increased risks of cardiovascular disorders including hypertension, gallbladder disease and diabetes. The prevention of dietary obesity depends on matching consumption of food to physiological requirements and its correction depends, therefore, on reducing intake or increasing exercise or both.

While it is generally accepted that the high sugar content of modern Western diets is conducive to obesity and dental caries, the importance of specific components of diet in pre-disposing to or causing disease is still the subject of wide debate. This centres particularly on the role of dietary fat in the aetiology of some diseases, notably heart disease and breast cancer, of salt in hypertension and of dietary fibre in cancer of the colon. The consumption of a diet high in saturated fats may lead to high serum lipid concentrations, particularly of low density lipoprotein cholesterol (LDLC). This is generally believed to be a major risk factor for development of coronary heart disease. Likewise high salt intake appears to predispose to hypertension. It has yet to be established by properly controlled trials that reversal of these risk factors by dietary means significantly reduces the incidence of these diseases. Similarly, although in some countries people who consume a diet low in fibre content have been shown to have higher incidence of cancer of the colon than those whose diet is rich in fibre, it is not certain that changing to a high fibre diet will reduce the risk. Despite these uncertainties the majority of informed opinion accepts that the balance of evidence now favours advising the public to make changes in their diet in the directions indicated by these findings.

The publication, in the early 1980s, of two authoritative reports, one by the Committee on Medical Aspects of Food Policy (COMA) and the other by the National Advisory Committee on Nutrition Education, confirmed these recommendations. The two reports received a great deal of publicity and related health education campaigns have encouraged a significant change in public attitudes and behaviour. The food industry has responded positively by providing, in supermarkets and elsewhere, a greatly improved range of low fat, reduced sugar and high fibre products. In addition, legal requirements on the labelling of food products enables the public to make more informed choices in the purchase of foods.

Chapter 15
Screening

Introduction

In some diseases the causes are complex and disease may be the result of hereditary factors or minimal exposure of susceptible individuals over long periods to causative agents whose nature and mode action may not be fully understood. Consequently, there are practical difficulties in applying the methods of prevention and control already outlined, such as the removal of the causal agent from the environment or enhancing host resistance by improved nutrition or the use of a vaccine. Likewise educating people in safe habits or behaviour is difficult when the cause of the disease is obscure. In such circumstances other approaches to control must be used. Intervention in the natural history of the disease itself is the most obvious alternative. Screening is the practice of investigating apparently healthy individuals with the object of detecting unrecognized disease or its precursors in order that measures can be taken that will prevent or delay the development of disease or improve the prognosis when it is already present. The rationale behind this approach is as follows.

In many diseases the pathological process is established long before the appearance of symptoms and signs which alert patients to the need to seek medical advice. By this time the disease process and the consequent damage may be irreversible, or difficult to treat. For example, in phenylketonuria, an inborn error of metabolism, the abnormality does not usually declare itself before irreversible brain damage has taken place. This can be averted if the condition is detected in the neonatal period and the affected infant is given a diet low in phenylalanine. In other diseases, patients with signs of disease, for example a woman with a lump in the breast or a person with impaired vision, may fail to consult a doctor because the symptoms are not sufficiently troublesome or because of fear or stoicism or for other reasons. It seems logical to believe that if potentially serious diseases were diagnosed and treated at an early stage many personal disasters might be averted. If so, then a programme aimed at their early detection would be a valuable preventive service.

In other diseases it may be possible to intervene at an even earlier stage in their natural history by treating precursor conditions, thereby reducing the risk that pathology will develop. For example, there is evidence that the risk of stroke can be reduced by controlling raised blood pressure, and that the risk of a woman developing invasive carcinoma of the cervix uteri may be reduced by the detection and treatment of carcinoma *in situ*. The recent introduction of mammographic screening for the detection of early breast cancer also rests on the same principle.

Lastly, it may be possible to identify individuals who are particularly vulnerable to disease, even though as yet no abnormality exists. Active intervention at this stage may reduce subsequent risk. For example, haemolytic disease of the newborn can be prevented by administration of anti-D antiserum to the rhesus negative mother of a rhesus positive fetus.

Another application of the screening principle is in the interests of the public health. Some individuals may be infected with an organism and, although they have no symptoms, are capable of transmitting it to other people. Such individuals are called carriers. The detection of the organism in such people will be of no benefit to them since they suffer no adverse consequences. However it is often in the interests of the people with whom they come in contact and the wider community that they should be identified. Ideally once identified they should be treated, but in some circumstances it is not possible to eliminate the organism; this has been the situation in the case of typhoid carriers. When treatment is not possible it may be advisable to isolate the affected individuals from situations that may be dangerous to others. For example, if there is an outbreak of penicillin resistant staphylococcus wound infections on a surgical unit it would be reasonable to screen all the operating theatre and ward staff in an attempt to identify the healthy carrier. Once identified that carrier would then be taken off clinical duties until such time as he or she was proven to be clear of infection. The wider application of screening in the interests of the public health (whether in an attempt to control the spread of disease or to understand the pathways by which it is spread) raises difficult ethical and moral issues. They are highlighted by the current concern regarding the spread of HIV. It could be argued that routine screening of certain groups might help in both understanding the dynamics of the transmission of HIV and in its control. On the other hand as there is no early treatment for HIV infection many believe that the pursuance of such a policy would represent an unreasonable and unacceptable intrusion on the privacy of individuals.

It should be noted that the use of screening in disease control involves some important assumptions. Some programmes, for example, rest on the assumption that a pathological process can be detected reliably before it is clinically manifest and that, if it is so detected, it can be reversed, arrested, retarded or alleviated more readily at this stage than if treatment were delayed until the patient presented with symptoms. For instance, the cervical cytology screening programme depends on two assumptions neither of which has ever been scientifically proven. The first of these is that carcinoma *in situ*, which is the condition which the screening process detects, commonly progresses to invasive carcinoma. The second is that invasive cervical carcinoma is invariably preceded by a phase of carcinoma *in situ*. If either of these assumptions is invalid the rationale of the programme fails. Moreover, it is impossible for obvious ethical reasons to carry out the long-term studies which would be required to test them.

Other types of screening procedures assume that people at high risk can be individually identified with reasonable accuracy and that intervention in their lives will avert or significantly reduce the likelihood that they will develop disease and disability. For example, screening for high levels of blood cholesterol is sometimes advocated on the assumption that if the cholesterol level can be reduced by dietary means then the person's riks of developing coronary heart disease will be reduced.

In certain circumstances screening is of undoubted benefit, for example antenatal screening, but good evidence of the value of many of the screening procedures which have gained popularity both with the medical profession and the public is, at present, lacking. Sometimes the early detection of disease serves only to extend the period of awareness that it is present without in any way improving the prognosis. Furthermore, in any screening programme, cases with a long and relatively benign natural history are more likely to be detected than those with a rapidly progressive and fatal outcome. The dividends from screening in these circumstances can be disappointing, unless the interval between successive examinations is carefully timed to take account of variations in the natural history of the disease in question.

Finally, before embarking on any screening programme it is necessary to remember three further important points.

1 In contrast to clinical practice which involves the patient *asking* for the doctor's aid to deal with established symptoms, in screening programmes apparently healthy people are *invited* to present themselves for examination. They have the right to assume that this will benefit them, or at least will do them no harm.

2 Screening large numbers of people is expensive and can divert both staff and financial resources from other health services activities. It is essential, therefore, to evaluate screening programmes adequately before they are introduced and to weigh the potential dividends both for the individuals screened and for the health of the community against the gains from alternative uses of the same resources, the so-called 'opportunity cost'.

3 In order to achieve their aim of reducing levels of morbidity and/or mortality from a particular disease, screening programmes require a high uptake rate, especially amongst particularly vulnerable groups. This is not always easy to achieve as has been found in cervical cytology screening where the most vulnerable groups—social classes IV and V—have the poorest uptake.

Screening programmes

There are two approaches to population screening programmes. One is to restrict screening to members of identifiable high risk groups in a population and the other is to attempt to include everyone at risk regardless of the degree of risk. Clearly it is more economical to focus screening programmes on high risk groups. Efforts can then be concentrated on securing high participation rates in order to maximize the yield of cases in relation to the effort and expense invested. Whole population screening is indicated only where it is impossible to define high risk groups with sufficient specificity and sensitivity to ensure that they include a high proportion of those likely to develop the disease. Even with so called 'mass screening' the programme will invariably be restricted to certain broad categories determined for example by age, sex, occupation or area of residence.

The two general types of screening programme are usually referred to as *selective screening* and *mass screening*. In either case the programme may be directed to the detection of a specific disease, 'single disease screening', or include a range of tests for a number of different conditions, 'multiphasic screening'.

Selective screening

Tests are used to detect a specific disease or predisposing condition in people who are known to be at high risk of having, or of developing, the condition.

Examples
Single disease screening:
    chest X-rays for evidence of pneumoconiosis in coal miners;
    amniocentesis for chromosomal abnormalities in the fetus in older women.
Multiphasic screening:
    antenatal examinations in pregnant women;
    pre-employment medical examinations in high risk occupational groups, e.g. nurses.

Mass screening

Large numbers of people are tested for the presence of disease or a predisposing condition without specific reference to their individual risk of having or developing the condition.

Examples
Single disease screening:
    tests for phenylketonuria and congenital dislocation of hip in infancy;
    cervical cytology for carcinoma in situ;
    mammography for breast carcinoma.
Multiphasic screening:
    biochemical profiles on hospital patients;
    routine health 'check up' (well woman clinics, pre-retirement groups, etc).

Criteria for screening programmes

Before the introduction of a screening programme certain criteria should be met. These can be considered under the following headings:
    importance of the disease;
    natural history of the disease;
    effectiveness of early treatment;
    availability and acceptability of treatment;
    characteristics of the test;
    acceptability of the test;
    population to be screened;
    cost of screening.

Importance of the disease

Diseases for which a screening programme is proposed should be important in respect of the seriousness of their consequences or their frequency or both. For example, despite its rarity, congenital hypothyroidism is undoubtedly worth detecting early both because of its serious consequences if untreated and because it is eminently treatable. At the other extreme, deafness in old people is a very common disability which is frequently caused by wax in the external canal, a trivial condition but easily treated with great benefit to the patient.

Natural history of the disease

The natural history of the disease must be known for two reasons. First, in order to identify the points at which the disease is potentially detectable by screening and at which active intervention is likely to be effective: this should be before irreversible damage has been done. Second, to enable the effects of any intervention to be evaluated. This information can only be derived from preliminary cohort studies.

The natural history of a disease is not necessarily the same in all people. In particular, diseases vary in the speed with which they progress at different ages. It is critical to a screening programme that the implications of this observation are understood. For example, if the interval between the first detectable pre-symptomic phase and the appearance of symptoms is less than the interval between screening tests, then cases will be missed. Within the same disease those cases with a long natural history, which by implication have the better prognosis, will be more likely to be detected than those with a short natural history. This variation is of critical importance when designing and evaluating a screening programme, e.g. for the early detection of breast cancer.

Effectiveness of early treatment

There is no value in detecting a disease early unless there is an effective treatment which improves the prognosis compared with treatment at a later stage. Consequently clinical trials of the proposed intervention are required, particularly because the frequency of spontaneous regression in the early stages of disease is often not known. The reversion of an observation in the presumed pathological range to one in the normal range must not be confused with successful treatment. Furthermore, treatments must be assessed in a group that is similar to that which it is proposed to screen. For example, if it is demonstrated that early treatment of mild hypertension reduces morbidity in a group of men aged 45–54 years, it cannot be assumed that it will benefit men aged 55–64 or 65–74 years who have similar blood pressures, nor that men in the 45–54 age group with higher biood pressures will enjoy the same improvement in prognosis.

It is essential to take great care to ensure that the comparison of early treatment (following pre-symptomatic screening) with treatment at a later stage is valid. Clearly early treatment will always increase survival time by at least the length of the interval between the pre-symptomatic diagnosis and symptomatic recognition: the so-called *lead time*. In estimating the true gain to the patients 'lead time' must be discounted.

Availability and acceptability of treatment

Clearly there is little point in the early detection of a disease unless the patient is willing to accept, and where appropriate, maintain treatment at this stage. When a patient has symptoms and believes that medical intervention will bring relief he or she is more likely to accept the treatment and even endure some side effects. In offering treatments in the absence of symptoms the doctor is in a difficult position. Long-term treatment for chronic disorders which cause no obvious and immediate disability, e.g. hypertension, may not always be successful because of non-compliance. This non-compliance may be because of a misunderstanding on the part of the patient, or because of unacceptable side effects or forgetfulness. Forgetfulness is probably the greatest problem as patients have no symptoms to remind them of their condition.

Sometimes delay in seeking medical aid may be because the patient is fearful of the disease itself or the treatment which he or she thinks may be offered. For example, some women may delay seeking advice about breast lumps because they perceive mastectomy as a more immediate and frightening prospect than the consequences of the disease, or because they see the diagnosis as a deferred but inevitable death sentence. In such cases the success of the screening programme will be limited.

Characteristics of the test

No screening programme is possible without a simple, safe and inexpensive test which can reliably detect predisposing conditions or the early stages of disease itself. The range of 'normal' findings by the test must be known. It should be quick to use because the object is to test large numbers of people. Unlike clinical practice in which a diagnosis and a decision to adopt a particular treatment is normally based on the history, the findings from physical examination and the results of laboratory investigations, screening is primarily a sorting process which depends on the results of a single test. This imposes particularly heavy demands on the test.

Tests are used to divide individuals who are screened into two groups—test positive and test negative. However, test positive does not always mean that the individual has the disease or predisposing condition and conversely test negative does not always mean that they are free from the disease or unlikely to contract it.

Conventionally the characteristics of a test are measured in terms of its *sensitivity* and *specificity* (see p. 37). In order to measure the sensitivity and specificity of a screening test it is desirable to conduct follow-up studies over a period of time amongst people who have been assigned to the positive or negative categories by the test but have not been treated. In some diseases the presumptive evidence of disease in test positive individuals is so strong and the potential consequences of failure to offer prompt treatment are so grave that it may be unethical to conduct such an investigation. However, if a screening programme is initiated without full knowledge of the test characteristics problems will arise. Although false negatives will become apparent in due course, these diminish the benefit to the community of the programme. Some of the false positives will be identified by subsequent investigations which precede definitive treatment but those that are not so identified and treated will tend to exaggerate the benefits of the programme. They will also waste resources.

The problems for patients of being falsely assigned to the positive category are that they may be subjected unnecessarily to time consuming, unpleasant and potentially harmful further investigations. Occasionally they may be submitted to unnecessary and harmful treatments. The false negative category presents different problems. Clearly the individuals concerned derive no benefit from the test itself. Furthermore, they may be falsely reassured that they are disease free, however carefully the test results are reported to them, and may delay seeking medical aid when symptoms subsequently appear.

Acceptability of the test

Much the same problems arise in relation to the acceptability of tests as in the acceptability of treatments. Symptomless patients are less amenable to uncomfortable, time-consuming and potentially dangerous investigations than those who are seeking medical aid for a problem or potential problem that they themselves recognize.

Population to be screened

Attention should be paid to the way in which individuals are recruited to a screening programme. Ideally all 'at risk' individuals should be identified and a systematic effort should be made to screen them all. This may be possible where relevant lists exist. For example, all newborn babies are known and can be screened for PKU. Those who respond to an 'open' invitation to attend for screening tend to come mainly from self selected 'health conscious' persons who are often those at least risk (low yield groups) but may also attract those who for one reason or another have delayed seeking advice about symptoms (high yield groups).

Cost of screening

Health services have to recognize that resources of all types are finite. The cost, including both direct and opportunity costs of a screening programme, must therefore be assessed before its introduction. The calculated cost of a screening programme to the health services should include the costs of all the screening tests performed (both manpower and consumables), the cost of further investigations to discriminate between the true and false positives, the total treatment costs of the positive cases, and the total treatment costs of the false negatives. The benefits include the savings on the treatment of cases if they had been allowed to present in the normal way, as well as the social benefits related to potentially lost earnings or the loss of a mother and the 'value' of pain and suffering that would have been incurred. These can be difficult to quantify.

It is of course unreasonable to initiate a screening programme unless there are sufficient resources (trained manpower, hospital beds, technical equipment, etc.) to meet the treatment needs identified by the programme.

Changes in any of the criteria that have been discussed here may alter the approach to the programme itself. It should therefore be perodically reassessed.

Part 3
Health Services

Chapter 16
History and Principles

Introduction

Health services fall into two broad categories:

1 personal health services;
2 public or environmental health services.

Personal health services include the whole range of preventive therapeutic and rehabilitative services provided for individuals. Public health services are concerned with the monitoring of disease and advice on the control of factors in the environment that may affect health. These include the quality and bacteriological safety of air, water, food, safe sewage disposal, the control of occupational and industrial hazards and environmental pollution, and the maintenance of housing standards. In a complex industrial society health may be affected by public policy in many fields that are not normally thought of as specifically 'health' services. Education, transport, housing, industrial, commercial and economic policies may all directly or indirectly influence the health and welfare of society. One of the functions of an effective public health service is to monitor these factors and to provide scientific evidence of their health implications.

The history and evolution of health services is described in this chapter. In Chapter 17 the present arrangements for the delivery of health services in England and Wales are described.

History of personal health services

One characteristic of Western societies is that they accept responsibility for the care of individuals who, through no fault of their own, are unable to care and provide for themselves. In general, these are the elderly, the poor, and the disabled. The most basic expression of this obligation to care is through the extended family, i.e. parents, siblings, children, uncles and aunts, together with others who identify with the family.

The main unit of rural societies is the family. Families normally live close together and share the same type of work. In these circumstances the personal caring aspect of the family's life is absorbed into its normal activities. In modern industrial societies, families are more mobile, both geographically and socially, and work is normally a separate activity from the day to day life. For this reason, even though the family may appreciate that it has a responsibility to those of its members who are unable to care for themselves, it is not in a position to assist them. For example, different generations may live in different towns, or the daytime job of the main wage earners of a nuclear family may preclude them from devoting sufficient time to the care of an aged relative. Moreover the role of women has changed from one of child bearer, child rearer and housekeeper to a partner in domestic matters and wage earning. Therefore, a service involving people other than the family has had to develop. The involvement of people outside the family in the care of people made it necessary to create a system for payment and generated the need for professional carers.

The process whereby personal health care evolved from being solely a family obligation to being a professional activity with state involvement in its financing and supervision was complex. It was influenced by the structure of societies, changes in the expectations of individuals and developments in medical science and technology leading to escalating costs.

In England the earliest legislation for the public provision of services for the sick was the Act for the Relief of the Poor (1598) usually referred to as the Poor Law, which required parishes to appoint an 'overseer of the poor . . . to raise money by local taxation and to provide . . . the necessary relief for the lame, impotent, old, blind and other such being poor and not able to work'. This legislation implicitly recognized the relationship between disablement and poverty and it restricted help to those who had no other source of support. In effect it was a last resort provision. It was not fully repealed until the passage of the NHS Act in 1946.

Early arrangements for the care of the sick were rudimentary. They were provided with shelter, food and basic attention. The roles of the doctors and of medicine were limited. During the twentieth century there has been dramatic progress in the development of medical skills and of medical technology. These have affected the shape of medical services in many ways. The new special skills and technologies had to be concentrated in institutions (hospitals) in order that they could develop. This brought about a change in the nature of the hospital from an institution concerned with the general care of the poor to one that was clearly medically orientated. Many people who whilst ill, had previously been looked after at home, turned to hospitals for investigation, care and treatment. Consequently the social mix of hospital patients changed and they ceased to be the last refuge of the neglected, the destitute and those whose families had dispersed. This changed the standards and nature of care offered within the hospitals.

Hospitals

Voluntary hospitals

A few hospitals were established in England by religious orders during the Middle Ages. These include St Bartholomew's and St Thomas's Hospitals in London. They were founded as practical demonstrations of Christian charity to provide care for the destitute. By 1700 there were fewer than 12 hospitals in the whole country, most of which were in London. The period during which the greatest amount of hospital building occurred was in the late eighteenth and early nineteenth centuries.

The voluntary hospitals were supported at first by church funds, charitable contributions and endowments. They were founded principally as places of asylum and rest for the physically sick and chronically disabled. They were staffed by unpaid doctors (consultants) and, in the teaching hospitals, by doctors in training. Their location was determined in part by local need and in part by the availability of 'private practice' for the honorary staff, which was their only source of income. Outside the main teaching centres there were other types of voluntary hospital, including cottage hospitals, funded locally and staffed by local general practitioners on a part-time basis.

The advent of more sophisticated medical treatments and diagnostic techniques—developed largely in the London teaching hospitals—made the voluntary hospitals become more selective in their admissions. They tended to admit patients whose stay was likely to be short and to avoid admitting the chronically sick. These were either admitted to or transferred to municipal hospitals.

By the end of the nineteenth century the clientele of the major voluntary hospitals were no longer limited to the destitute. Because of the increasing costs of providing a service, they had to introduce a system of payment for those who could afford to pay. The charitable funds were used for those who could not. Most hospitals employed 'lady almoners' whose job it was to establish who should be subsidised and to what extent. Despite the introduction of a semi fee-paying system, the costs of maintaining these hospitals rose faster than their incomes fell and they became increasingly financially embarrassed.

At the outbreak of World War II the government set up the Emergency Medical Service in order to meet the large number of military and civilian casualties that were expected. This guaranteed money to the voluntary hospitals to meet the predicted need. After the war lack of a secure income made a return to their former independent status impossible. Most of them became part of the National Health Service in 1948.

Municipal hospitals

The Elizabethan Poor Law enabled parishes to attach infirmary wards to workhouses. Parishes were small population units and in order to produce a viable system groups of parishes combined to administer the Poor Law legislation. These groups were called Parish Unions. Boards of Guardians were responsible for the day to day administration of the institutions.

The poor Law infirmaries were for the destitute sick and were quite unlike hospitals as we know them today. At first they did not have any medical staff: nursing care was provided by the non-sick inmates of the workhouse. Over the years the infirmaries improved, although there was considerable variation in standards.

A feature of much of the Poor Law legislation and the legislation governing matters of public health was that although it gave local authorities discretionary powers to improve the standards and scope of care, it did not place a duty on them to do so. In this lies one of the reasons for the present maldistribution of health care resources in Britain. The Poor Law infirmaries were made over to local government authorities in 1929. They then became municipal hospitals. From then until the outbreak of World War II a concerted effort was made to improve standards and staffing. In 1939 the municipal hospitals were grouped with the voluntary hospitals in regions as part of the Emergency Medical Service.

Other hospitals

There were two other types of public hospitals during the first half of the twentieth century—fever hospitals and lunatic asylums.

The fever hospitals were established to protect the public from infection. Only later were they able to offer treatment. Among them were large numbers of tuberculosis sanitoria. They were built between the two World Wars and are testaments to the high prevalence of that disease and to increasing faith in its treatment.

The lunatic asylums had a chequered history. Until 1890 the mentally disturbed were cared for in private mad houses (some with appalling reputations) or in prison or in workhouses (not the workhouse infirmary which was established for the physically sick).

The Lunacy Act of 1890 placed a duty on county authorities to provide asylums for those of unsound mind. The London County Council built many such hospitals including nine, with accommodation for several thousand patients, around Epsom in Surrey. The distance from London did not deter the planners as they took it for granted that once patients were admitted there was little chance that they would ever be discharged.

The medical profession

Doctors

Until the middle of the nineteenth century there were three types of medical men:

> physicians;
> surgeons;
> apothecaries.

Nearly all of these worked almost entirely outside hospitals.

Physicians

These were university graduates (mainly from Oxford and Cambridge) who had then qualified for a diploma of the Royal College of Physicians (founded in 1518). Their background was upper class and their practice was mainly among the upper and merchant classes. They attended the voluntary hospitals on a charitable basis.

Surgeons

These qualified with a diploma from the Royal College of Surgeons (founded in 1800). They frequently worked under the supervision of the physicians.

Apothecaries

The third group of medical men, who co-existed with the physicians and surgeons, were the Apothecaries. Strictly, they were apprentice-trained tradesmen whose qualification was in making medicines rather than in diagnosis and prescribing. Although they did act as doctors, they were breaking the law in pursuing such activities. They extended their activities during the plague when most physicians left London along with other members of the upper classes. Then, by default, the apothecaries adopted a new role. By the beginning of the nineteenth century the apothecaries were well established as doctors to all but the upper classes. They were not, however, appointed to the honorary staff of the voluntary hospitals.

The General Medical Council

In 1853, physicians, surgeons and apothecaries were placed on a common register maintained by the General Medical Council which was charged with control over their training and qualifications. Specialities developed in the hospitals because of the facilities offered there, while the doctors who worked mainly in the community became known as general practitioners. In the growing connurbations the fact that people could be seen free of charge in the out-patient departments of the voluntary hospitals caused some resentment among general practitioners. In order to overcome this, a system was developed whereby patients would only be seen in out-patients if referred by their regular doctor.

Domiciliary health services

General practice

By 1909, while out-patients at hospital could normally be seen free of charge after referral, the majority of the population paid their general practitioner a fee for consultation. A small number of *provident societies* were been established to which people could subscribe to ensure that money was available to pay doctors' bills. The boards of guardians provided a rudimentary domiciliary service to the very poor.

National Health Insurance Act

The Poor Law Commission (1909) demonstrated that a lack of early medical advice often resulted in prolonged sickness and consequent poverty. In 1911 Lloyd George's National Health Insurance Act became law. Its important provisions were:
- Weekly payments to insured persons while sick to enable them to maintain minimal living standards.
- Free medical treatment from a general practitioner who the insured person was free to choose (provided the doctor had agreed to participate in the scheme).
- Doctors who participated in the scheme were paid on a capitation basis, i.e. so much per year per person registered. This was advantageous to the general practitioner as it guaranteed him a regular income for the first time.

The scheme was restricted to working men whose income was below a specified minimum amount. It did not include retired persons, the wives of working men or their children. The scheme was administered by approved friendly societies.

In subsequent years the National Insurance scheme was extended and, by 1945, the majority of the population was covered.

Domiciliary nursing

At the beginning of the nineteenth century there were few trained nurses. The need for home nursing was appreciated by the middle of the century and in 1887 the Queen's Institute of District Nursing was established. This institute maintained standards of practice and coordinated local voluntary committees.

Mothers and infants

The extremely high maternal and infant mortality in the nineteenth century led social reformers to look for ways of preventing this waste of life. Important landmarks are:

Foundation of the Manchester and Salford Sanitary Association, 1862
This organization employed women to give instruction and guidance to mothers on child rearing. The scheme eventually developed into what is now known as Health Visiting.

The Midwives Act, 1902
This prohibited untrained women from practising midwifery.

The Maternity and Child Welfare Act, 1918
This obliged local authorities to provide a medical service for expectant mothers, nursing mothers and children under 5 years of age.

The Midwives Act, 1936
This made local authorities responsible for ensuring that there were sufficient midwives to meet the population's need.

The present tasks of personal medical services

The changes in medical practice during the past 50 years have been revolutionary. Today access to complex technology, skilled personnel and powerful therapies is taken for granted. Some illnesses that were inaccessible to medical intervention a generation ago, can now be treated by methods that are now commonplace. In all branches of medicine there remains a need for the traditional role of the doctor, that of an informed professional carer rather than a medical scientist who is always expected to cure. In some cases medicine still has little to offer other than palliation and understanding; in others once the correct diagnosis has been made the doctor's role is simply one of supervising long-term treatment. Often the tasks of medicine are submerged in the administrative structure of health services. It is useful to consider the range of basic types of provision that are essential to a comprehensive health service.

Fortunately most of the population is fit and well for most of the time; they will only require access to medicine when they become sick. Broadly the sick can be divided into those who require access to the modern technology of medicine both for the investigation and treatment of their illnesses and those for whom such facilities are less important than access to carers who have a thorough understanding of them as people and the effects the illness is having upon them. It follows that a modern health service must provide facilities that are accessible to everyone who becomes sick and appropriate services for the chronic sick.

Primary care

Primary care services are required for the whole population. They should enable individuals who become ill, or think they have a medical problem, to obtain advice, treatment or sometimes referral to a specialist service. Primary care services are provided in general practice, occupational health services, accident and emergency departments, first aid rooms and many other places. The precise location of primary care varies from country to country: in most societies there are many alternative sources of such care.

Secondary care

Secondary care for those who require access to the technology of medicine is almost universally provided within a hospital. In the UK, hospitals designed for this purpose are called acute hospitals; in other countries other terms, e.g. somatic hospital, are used but the activities that occur within them are the same. Medical care that is dependent upon technology is concentrated in hospitals in order to reduce the cost of equipment and to retain the skill of personnel which would otherwise decline through lack of practice. The task of acute hospitals is to diagnose, to initiate treatment and, when the equipment to treat is only available at the hospital, to complete the course of treatment. It is not their role to accumulate patients or to provide long-term care for people who do not require their facilities. In planning terms the location of an acute hospital is less important than the location of an institution that provides long-term care and support because it is assumed that the patients will require the acute facilities for a relatively short period.

Another type of secondary care is required for long-term sick and those who do not require the facilities of a modern hospital. Ideally this should be provided as close to the residence of the patients as possible. Sometimes it is feasible to provide it at home. Much of the work of general practice falls into this category and most of this type of care is in fact provided by general practitioners. About 80% of the consultations (whether in the surgery or at the patients home) of general practitioners are generated by about 20% of the population. A large proportion of that 20% are the chronic sick and depend entirely on the general practitioner and his primary care team for their medical care. There are other sources of secondary care that do not depend upon technology. These include psychiatric units, hospitals and institutions for the mentally handicapped, geriatric hospitals, hospices for the dying, homes for the young chronic sick and centres for those disabled by serious permanent injury or disease. In most cases the decision to provide long-term care in a specialist institution rather than in their own home is affected more by the social circumstances and the availability of the family and friends to provide basic support than it is by the patient's medical condition.

Personal health care services must include easy access to preventive medicine (immunization, screening, health education, etc). This is provided in a variety of ways including mother and child clinics, school clinics, well-women clinics, occupational health centres and general practice. In the absence of such resources many avoidable illnesses will occur to the disadvantage of the individuals and society as a whole.

It is clear that the role of the general practitioner is very broad but few of his activities are exclusive to him. It is also clear that the most expensive areas in the provision of medical care are the acute hospitals. It is unlikely that any society will achieve the ideal balance in its provision of services and there will always be a need to modify provision in the light of the circumstances of a society. In general the rich countries of the world can afford the luxury of the expensive technology but the poorer developing countries of the Third World must concentrate their sparse resources on personal preventive services, primary care and secondary care that is not dependent on the most modern, and expensive medical technology.

Public Health Service

The involvement of the State in the provision and financing of health services arose from increasing public acceptance of the obligation of the community to bear collective responsibility for the health and welfare of its members. Moreover, as the development of medical science in the nineteenth century, particularly in the field of microbiology, began to uncover the causes of the major infectious diseases, including typhoid, cholera and smallpox which ravaged the rapidly growing cities of the industrial revolution it became clear, first that these plagues were preventable and, second, that their prevention could only be achieved by state action. Such action was essential both to provide the physical infrastructure which could ensure a bacteriologically safe water supply and safe disposal of sewage, and also to establish the means of monitoring and enforcing adequate environmental control.

Appreciation of these facts led to the growth of the Public Health Movement in the mid-century. The main thrust of this was directed to sanitary reform measures backed by appropriate legislation. The Nuisances Removal Act (1846) gave local authorities power to clean up the towns, though it did not require them to do so. The first Public Health Act was passed in 1848 in the wake of a disastrous outbreak of cholera. This set up a General Board of Health with local boards to be responsible for the improvements outlined in the 1848 Act.

The next major Public Health Act of 1875 obliged local authorities to improve provisions for disposal of sewage, to provide pure water supplies and street cleaning, to improve housing standards, and many other aspects of town life. The authorities were also then *obliged* to appoint Medical Officers of Health to advise them on matters relating to the health of the community. Interestingly, occupational health services were not included in this legislation and remain outside the National Health Service to the present day.

When local authorities were established in their modern form in the nineteenth century their principal role was to administer environmental health services. Despite having acquired over the years a vast range of other functions, they continue via their Environmental Health Departments, with their staff of well-trained environmental health officers, to be the principal local agencies responsible for monitoring and enforcing environmental standards relating to food, water supplies and sewage disposal, air quality, housing, and working conditions other than in factories (which are the responsibility of the Health and Safety Executive), etc. They also carry statutory responsibility for the investigation and control of communicable disease in the community, obtaining medical advice for this and other purposes from doctors (consultants in public health medicine) employed by the corresponding district health authority.

The Ministry of Health was created in 1919 to exert more effective control over local bodies in the field of preventive health. The last important Public Health Act before the National Health Service was passed in 1936. It codified and simplified practice relating to environmental and personal hygiene. Thus, by 1947, public environmental health practice and its administration had evolved a structure close to its modern pattern, although it remained separate from facilities for the treatment of the sick.

Doctors have played a crucial role in the development of public health services from the time of the appointment of the first Medical Officer of Health (MOH) in Liverpool in 1847. The 1875 Public Health Act obliged all local authorities to appoint an MOH whose main responsibilities were to advise the local authority on matters related to environmental health. Over the next 50 years this cadre of doctors who specialized in public health grew and the scope of their work enlarged to embrace many personal preventative services such as the school health service, maternity and child welfare, immunization, health education, social support services for the elderly, mentally ill and disabled, and some treatment services (e.g. tuberculosis and venereal diseases). In 1974 the Medical Officers of Health and their personal health service responsibilities were brought into the NHS. At the same time, they, together with doctors working in medical administration and in relevant university departments, came together to form the new specialty of community medicine. A recent report, *Public health in England* (1988), has recommended a return to the old title of public health medicine and doctors specializing in this field are now called public health physicians. The report also re-defines their role: in essence this is to enquire into all matters which affect the health of communities or population groups, to measure health care needs, to plan, administer and evaluate services, with particular reference to the prevention of disease and promotion of health in the community, and to provide relevant advice to health authorities, central Government and other bodies.

Chapter 17
The National Health Service

Origins of the National Health Service

The important report by Sir William Beveridge on social and allied services, published in 1942 was the culmination of many years of pressure for social reform. It recommended that the State should finance and provide a comprehensive social security system and that it should be underpinned by a comprehensive national health service. It specifically proposed that a National Health Service should provide the facilities which would:

> ... ensure that for every citizen there is available whatever medical treatment he requires in whatever form he requires it, domiciliary or institutional, general, specialist or consultant, and will ensure also the provision of dental, ophthalmic and surgical appliances, nursing and midwifery, and rehabilitation after accidents.

Apart from humanitarian considerations, which were the principal motivations for the proposals, Beveridge made the apparently hard headed assertion that such a health service would reduce the costs of social security payments by decreasing the amount of illness in the population. It was thought that this would increase the general appeal of the proposals.

When estimating the possible costs of a health service, Beveridge and his colleagues made the further, and, as it turned out, disastrously naive assumption. They assumed that, as the health of the population improved because of the abolition of poverty, better preventive medicine and the elimination of the long-standing pool of untreated chronic illness, the cost of the proposed National Health Service would diminish. They failed to take account of the possibility that changes in the expectations of the public in the level of health care, the consequences of an ageing population and changes in the costs of medical technology and of manpower might invalidate many of the costing assumptions. Time has proved his assumptions to be wrong.

The wartime coalition government accepted the general proposal for comprehensive national social security and health care systems but was unable to implement them immediately. It charged the Minister of Health for England and Wales, and Secretary of State for Scotland with the responsibility of initiating consultations with representatives of the medical profession, the voluntary hospitals, and the local authorities. Discussions began early in 1943 and on 8 February 1944 a White Paper on 'The National Health Service' (Cmd. 6502) was published. Its stated objective was:

> ... to show what is meant by a comprehensive service and how it fits with what has been done in the past, or is being done in the present, and so help people to look at the matter for themselves.

The publication of the White Paper served to crystallize ideas and to stimulate criticism. By the end of 1944 the Minister of Health submitted the suggestions that he had received from all interested parties to the Government. Basically the proposals involved the government taking financial and other responsibility for the municipal, voluntary and other hospitals, for the general practitioner services as set up under the 1911 Act, and for municipal public health services and other aspects of personal and preventive medical services. Access to all services was to be without direct charges at the time of use for all residents of the country. In essence the availability of the then existing services was to be extended but their basic philosophy and administration changed little. On 19 March 1946 a Bill providing for the establishment of a comprehensive health service was presented to Parliament. Royal Assent was given to the National Health Service Act on 6 November 1946 and the Service was launched in 1948.

The National Health Service 1948

The administration of original health service was divided into:
hospital services;
general practitioner services;
local authority services.

Hospital services

Fourteen Regional Hospital Boards were established within which there were 290 Hospital Groups each administered by a Hospital Management Committee. The teaching hospitals (both undergraduate and postgraduate) were autonomous from the Regional Hospital Boards. Each had their own Boards of Governors which worked in close cooperation with the governing body of the associated university institution.

General practitioner services

The administration of general medical services was the responsibility of 134 Executive Councils. They administered:
general medical services (family doctors);
general dental services;
pharmaceutical services;
ophthalmic services.

All of the above services were, and still are, provided on an independent contractual basis. This means that the doctors, dentists, opticians, ophthalmic medical practitioners and pharmacists are not employed by the NHS; they are paid by the NHS for the actual services provided. The Executive Councils had limited disciplinary and planning functions, their main role was that of a paying body. Technically, general practitioners and other independent contractors were directly accountable to the Minister. In effect the contractual position of this group of practitioners was little different to that under the 1911 legislation.

Local authority services

The local government authorities were responsible for the care and after care of patients in the community and with the prevention of ill health. Specifically they were responsible for:

antenatal care;

midwifery;

infant and child welfare;

district (domiciliary) nursing;

health visiting;

school health services;

immunization;

ambulance services;

environmental health and a number of other functions relating to the control of infectious disease.

Early problems

In its early years the National Health Service experienced many difficulties and shortcomings. The most important of these were:

• There had been a gross underestimate of cost. Demand increased as new services were provided. The estimated first year cost of the National Health Service was £179 million. It actually cost £400 million.

• The National Health Service inherited many old and small hospitals, which had been built under the Poor Law provisions. After the war the Government's first priority was to build houses rather than hospitals. As a result there was almost no new hospital building for the first 20 years of the existence of the NHS.

• The division of administration of the service between three bodies (hospitals, general practitioners and public health) resulted in lack of coordination and cooperation. For example, many hospitals served several different local authority areas: and all three divisions of the service were involved in maternity services.

• The NHS had failed to correct the long-standing inequalities in service provision between different parts of the country and between different types of service. The most neglected services were the care of the aged and mentally ill together with services for the chronic sick and disabled. The northern regions of the country were poorly provided with hospitals but the areas in and around London had a historical over provision. The continued geographical mal-distribution of facilities was at least partly due to the fact that there was inadequate capital investment in new hospitals in those regions that had a long-standing historical under provision.

Changes in the 1960s and 1970s

The original tripartite structure of the NHS was seen as a hindrance to the achievement of an integrated and balanced service throughout the country. As a result of a series of enquiries and reports by advisory groups in the 1960s a major reorganization of the NHS occurred in 1974. The most important aspects of that reorganization were that the country was divided into a number of Regional Health Authorities (RHAs) within each of which there were a number of Area Health Authorities (AHAs) each of which was subdivided into two or more Districts (DHAs). The authorities were responsible for the provision of all services other than the independent contractor services within their defined geographical boundaries. As far as was possible the geographical boundaries of the health authorities were the same as those of the local government authorities. The independent contractors (general medical practice, general dental practice, pharmaceutical service, ophthalmic services, etc) were the responsibility of Family Practitioner Committees. The RHAs had a mainly strategic planning and financial control role; the AHAs planned and managed some of the services whilst the Districts were responsible for the day to day management of services.

In 1982 the AHAs were abolished. Some of their responsibilities were transferred to the RHAs and other to the districts—which became authorities in their own right. In 1984 there was a further reorganization that was designed to make the decision making in the service and its financial control more efficient by the introduction of general management.

The present management arrangements

The principles which currently govern the management of the service are that the health authorities are responsible for planning and managing all state health services within specified geographical areas and that, within general strategies and financial limits they have considerable autonomy to allow them to respond to local needs. The general strategies and financial allocations are decided by government and the NHS Management Board. These are acted upon by the RHAs and generally implemented by the DHAs.

The *Secretary of State for Health* is responsible to Parliament for the NHS. He is a member of the Cabinet and, as such, he is able to bring the needs of the Service to the attention of his colleagues and to argue the case for the money required for the service. He is also responsible for the enactment of government policy on health matters. He must account to Parliament for the expenditure of the Service and for its performance. He is assisted by two Ministers for Health.

The *DoH* provides the administrative support to the Secretary of State and his Ministers. Its main functions are to assist ministers by supplying them with the information they need regarding the working of the service, to advise them on the choices available when making policy decisions and the possible consequences of the available options, to transmit policy decisions to the regions, and monitor progress in their achievement.

In addition to the section of the department which is directly concerned with the day to day work of Ministers, the department is divided into the following main divisions. These deal respectively with:

regional liaison matters;

NHS manpower;

NHS finance;

NHS support services (building design, maintenance, equipment, etc).

Regional Health Authorities

There are 14 RHAs in England. Each serves populations of between 2.5 and 4.5 million. Each authority has between 17 and 25 members and a chairman. The chairman and all of the members of the RHAs are appointed by and accountable to the Secretary of State. Although the Secretary of State is obliged to consult a wide range of organizations before appointing authority members, including local authorities, universities, professional bodies, trades unions, etc, the individual members are appointed in their own right they are not representatives of any particular group or interest.

The chief executive of the RHA is the Regional General Manager and he has the ultimate responsibility to the authority for the management of the service and for the advice given to the authority by the permanent staff of the region. He is normally supported by a number of senior officers including Directors of Public Health, Finance, Estate Management and Planning.

The RHAs are broadly responsible for strategic (long-term) planning within their regions and for the provision of some services. The types of function that they perform include:

planning and policy making;
allocation of financial and other resources between districts within the region;
monitoring the performance and efficiency of the districts;
regional personnel policies and training;
major capital building and supply programmes in the region;
management of property;
provision of ambulance services, blood transfusion services, information services, public relations and legal services;
employment of certain staff including some consultant medical staff and senior registrars.

District Health Authorities

Each of the regions is divided into a number of DHAs. At present there are approximately 190 DHAs serving populations ranging from 100 000 to 900 000, the majority cover populations of around 250 000. The chairman of the authority is appointed by the Secretary of State. Some members of the authority are appointed by the RHA after consultation with local bodies with an interest in the service or consultation with professional organizations. Others are appointed by the local authorities within the boundaries of the DHA.

The DHA is responsible for the planning and management of all health services within its boundaries in accordance with the strategic guidelines and financial limits laid down by its RHA. In recognized teaching districts, normally districts in which there is a medical school, the authority has to discharge the Secretary of State's obligation to provide the necessary facilities for the training of university undergraduates and postgraduates.

The chief executive of the DHA is the District General Manager. He is responsible to the authority for the performance of the service and advises them on planning and strategic matters. He also liaises closely with the permanent staff of the RHA in order to advise them of the local situation and be appraised of their medium and long-term plans. He is supported by two or more Unit Managers (for the hospitals, community services, etc) and District Directors of Public Health, Finance, Planning, Personnel, Information and Information Technology. Within each of the districts there are a series of advisory committees, e.g. medical, nursing, etc. The District General Manager does not have to consult the advisory committees within the district before making a management decision nor does he have to accept any of the advice that he is given.

Services Managed by the District Health Authority

Acute hospital services

Most districts have at least one district general hospital. Normally all of the so-called 'district specialities', except those which the authority has arranged for other authorities to provide, are represented in these hospitals. Residents of the district are not obliged to use the hospital within their district. They or their general practitioner may feel that another hospital is preferable, either due to ease of access or because of the facilities offered. Although there is considerable referral to hospitals outside the district of residence, with the exception of the large urban connurbation there is rarely a net inflow of patients to or outflow from the district for hospital treatments.

The 'district specialities' include general medicine, general surgery, ortho-paedics, ENT, obstetrics and gynaecology, ophthalmology and paediatrics. Some district hospitals also provide regional speciality facilities. These are specialities where referral is from consultant to consultant, e.g. radiotherapy, cardiology, cardiac surgery, neurology, neurosurgery, rather than specialties to which the general practitioner refers directly.

The day to day management of hospitals is the responsibility of Unit General Managers who are supported by a team of other managers with responsibilities for discrete areas, e.g. hotel services, nursing services, outpatients services, etc.

Geriatric services

Districts provide both acute and long-stay geriatric facilities. Sometimes the acute geriatric services are provided in the district general hospital, in which they are often part of the day to day work of the general physicians. Although it is thought desirable to integrate chronic hospital geriatric care with the mainstream of hospital care it is often provided in separate long-stay institutions. Proper geriatric care involves the integration of the services in the hospital with those in the community and therefore in many districts the long-stay geriatric units form part of the responsibilities of the Community Unit Manager.

District nursing and health visitor services

The district has to provide adequate district nursing services to assist general practitioners to provide proper care to people in their own homes. The principal activities of district nurses are in the care of patients following discharge from hospital and in the long-term care of the elderly chronic sick. Health visitors are nurses who have had additional training in preventive medicine and health education. They are mainly concerned with giving advice and help regarding the health of infants and children and with preventive care amongst the elderly. There has been a trend towards the integration of district nurses and health visitors with general practitioners and members of other caring professions to form the primary care team. These services are the responsibility of the Community Unit Manager.

Obstetric services

The provision of obstetric services is the responsibility of the DHA. They include antenatal care, in-patient facilities for the care of pregnant women and delivery of their babies, postnatal care and domiciliary midwifery services.

Mental illness

The care of the mentally ill requires the provision of facilities, both short and long-stay (which constitute the bulk of the mentally ill), community psychiatric nurses and day hospital care. These are the responsibility of the Mental Health Unit Manager.

Mental handicap

Although about half the people with mental handicaps live in long-stay hospitals that are administered by the DHAs, there are large numbers in the community whose care is provided by the staffs of the health and local authorities. Most districts have one or more special teams that liaise closely with the social services staff, educational authorities and voluntary organizations in order to plan and provide adequate services for this group.

Health centres

Health centre provision is a responsibility of the DHAs. A health centre is designed to accommodate the community nurses, health visitors, chiropodists, etc and to offer accommodation to general practitioners.

Social workers

Social workers are *not* employed by the DHAs, they are employed by the social service departments of the local authorities. The DHA has to provide facilities for them to work in hospitals where they have an invaluable role in giving advice and making social services available to the sick.

Family Practitioner Committees

The Family Practitioner Committees (FPCs) are responsible for the supervision of services provided for the NHS by independent practitioners in contract with them to provide services. These are general practitioners, general dental practitioners, ophthalmic and dispensing opticians and pharmaceutical contractors. None of these is employed by the NHS, each is in contract with the NHS through the FPC to provide specified services and they are paid for the work they do. Thus the pharmaceutical chemist is paid for the drugs he dispenses plus a fee for dispensing, a general dental practitioner is paid by item of service, a general practitioner is paid in part by capitation, in part by item of service and some of his expenses are reimbursed. The areas covered by the FPC often include more than one DHA. The DHA consults the FPC when planning such developments as health centres.

Each FPC has 30 members who are appointed so as to include representative of the DHAs, the relevant local authorities, the Local Medical Committee (the local professional organization of general practitioners), the Local Dental Committee, the Local Pharmaceutical Committee, ophthalmic opticians and dispensing opticians. There are a number of 'lay' members.

The FPC elects its own chairman and has a full-time manager with a large clerical staff.

Local Medical Committees are comprised of general practitioners elected by their colleagues. Their role is to advise the FPC. Local dental and pharmaceutical committees have corresponding functions.

Community Health Councils

These are set up by the RHA to represent the interests of the public in health service matters. Their membership comprises representatives of local voluntary organizations concerned with health and members of the local authority. Although they are statutory bodies they do not have an executive role. They have certain rights of access of health service premises and to information relevant to their role. They also have the right to comment on the DHA's plans and to make alternative proposals which the DHA is obliged to consider.

The cost of the National Health Service

Sources of finance

All employed persons in the UK pay compulsory weekly or monthly national insurance contributions which partly finance the NHS. However, the major proportion of the cost of the NHS is met from central government funds, that is from general taxation. Other finance comes from charges to users, these include dental charges, prescription charges and charges to private patients in NHS hospitals (Table 17.1). The level of charges to users and the income they

Table 17.1 Sources of finance of the National Health Service (England).

	1976/77		1986/87	
	£1 000 000	Percentage of total income	£1 000 000	Percentage of total income
Consolidated funds (general taxation)	4532	87.6	13213	83.7
NHS contributions	518	10.0	1918	12.1
Charges to recipients	114	2.2	485	3.1
Miscellaneous	10	0.2	178	1.1
Total	5174	100.0	15794	100.0

yield varies from time to time. In 1986/7 the total expenditure on the NHS amounted to between 5 and 6% of the gross national product.

Expenditure

The main categories of expenditure are shown in Table 17.2. Central administration costs are mainly incurred by the DoH. The expenditure of the health authorities includes the costs of all types of hospital, community services, ambulance services, preventive medicine, health education, domiciliary nursing and health visiting and all the other provisions outlined above.

Hospitals

Expenditure on hospitals falls into two types:
    capital (new building and equipment);
    current (maintenance, wages and salaries, etc).

Hospital capital expenditure

Most of this expenditure is used to build new hospitals and major refurbishments of old hospital building. As it takes up to 10 years to plan and build a large new hospital, the annual amount of money spent on capital projects is a poor indicator of the commitment to the future improvement of facilities. The NHS suffers from the fact that many of the hospitals currently in use were built in the nineteenth century. They present many problems, including the following.

Table 17.2 Costs of the National Health Services 1986/87.

	£1 000 000	Percentage of total income
Central administration	135	0.89
Health Authorities		
Capital	936	5.95
Hospital services revenue	8256	52.51
Community services revenue	1055	6.71
Other services	573	3.64
Administration	435	2.77
Family Practitioner Committees		
Administration	95	0.06
General medical	1131	7.19
Pharmaceutical	1816	11.55
General dental	744	4.73
General ophthalmic	129	0.82
Other	417	2.65
Total	15722	100

Siting

Populations have increased in some areas while other areas have been depopulated since the hospitals were built. Central London, for instance, has many more hospitals than would be justified by its present resident population, although they now have major national specialist and training functions.

Mental hospitals tended to be built outside the population centres and some are still located at great distances from the communities they serve.

Design

The design of the institutions is often incompatible with the needs of modern medicine. Two particular examples are important:

- Many acute hospitals are ill-adapted to the needs of high technology medicine
- Long-stay hospitals are housed in old buildings, often with large long-stay wards with few or no day facilities.

Maintenance

Old buildings are expensive to maintain. This expenditure is not always rewarding because the basic design is inappropriate.

Hospital current expenditure

About 65% of the total hospital revenue expenditure is on wages and salaries. This leaves little room for financial manoeuvre because the numbers of doctors, nurses and other professional staff cannot easily be adjusted to short-term changes in need, and cuts in this direction usually lead to a decline in services. Table 17.3 shows the estimated cost per in-patient week for different types of hospitals. The differences between the costs of hospitals of different types is substantially due to variations in the numbers of staff that are required to provide the services required by patients admitted to such bed. This includes the clinical staff directly involved in the care of the patient and the specialist and technical staff who are required to enable the clinicians to function adequately (radiologists, pathologists, radiographers, scientists, laboratory technicians, operating theatre staff, intensive care staff, etc). There are also differences between

Table 17.3 Estimated average cost per in-patient week 1986/87.

	£
Teaching hospitals (acute)	
London	937.37
Outside London	806.40
Non-teaching hospitals	
Acute	712.73
Mainly acute	601.44
Geriatric	311.43
Maternity	781.90
Mental illness	308.35
Mental handicap	273.35

hospitals of different types in the amount of capital investment required in instruments and machinery. As manpower accounts for the major proportion of hospital costs, the weekly costs are only marginally affected by whether or not a bed is occupied or the appropriateness of its use. Thus a chronically sick person being cared for in an acute bed will cost almost the same as an acutely sick person in the same bed.

Family practitioner services

General practice

General practitioners are paid on a capitation basis (a fixed amount per year for each of the patients registered with them), supplemented by other payments including basic allowances, fees for items of service and reimbursments for approved expenses. The FPC has little budgetary control over the monies that it disburses.

Pharmaceutical services

The FPC expenditure on pharmaceutical services does not include the costs of drugs prescribed by hospitals, whether to in-patients or to out-patients. General practitioners write prescriptions on approved forms (FP10). These are taken by the patient or his representative to a pharmacist where they are dispensed (except in some rural areas where the general practitioner dispenses his own prescriptions). There are about 11 000 pharmaceutical contractors with the NHS (one for every two general practitioners). About 322.6 million prescriptions are dispensed annually. It should be noted that the amount of money spent on the drugs prescribed by general practitioners exceeds the total amount of money spent on the provision of general practice services. Table 17.4 shows the total net cost of prescriptions and the average number of prescriptions per year for different types of drugs.

The total cost of different types of drugs to the NHS is affected by the basic cost of the product and the prevalence of the disease that is being treated. Although the average cost of a prescription of a drug for the treatment of malignant disease is high (£26.71) (1990 price) the contribution of drugs used for the treatment of malignant disease to the NHS drug bill is very small—this is because malignant disease is relatively uncommon. By contrast the contribution of drugs for the treatment of disorders of the nervous system to the total drugs bill is high although the average cost per prescription is low—this is consistent with the very high incidence of treatments of disorders of the nervous system, especially the neurotic symptoms with tranquilizers and antidepressants.

Planning health services

Objectives

The health service has no single and easily definable objective. Various facilities are provided, including specialist services for the acute sick, preventive services, primary care and care for the chronic sick and disabled. Most of the work

Table 17.4 Total cost, average prescription cost and average number of prescriptions of different types in England, 1986.

Prescriptions for drugs acting on:	Total cost (£1 000 000)	Average cost per prescription (£)	Prescription per person per year
Nervous system	148	2.31	1.35
Hypnotics	20	1.54	0.27
Tranquillizers	14	1.25	0.24
Analgesics	25	1.51	0.35
Antidepressants	26	3.93	0.14
Gastrointestinal system	144	6.08	0.05
Antacids	6	1.50	0.08
Cardiovascular system	324	5.69	1.21
Heart	150	6.56	0.48
Diuretics	60	2.78	0.45
Antihypertensives	79	9.75	0.17
Respiratory system	129	4.33	0.63
Treatment of asthma	115	5.75	0.42
Rheumatism	169	8.89	0.40
Infections	131	3.20	0.87
Hormones	86	4.91	0.37
Haemopoesis	9	1.35	0.12
Malignant disease	16	26.71	0.01
Skin	78	3.51	0.47
Total	1366	4.23	6.83

involving direct intervention in acute sickness is purely medical in content, that is, it is mainly dependent upon the technical skills of doctors, often supported by the other highly trained staff. The care of the chronic sick requires the skill of others, such as nurses and social workers, as well as those of doctors. Many preventive programmes require action by non-medical professionals, e.g. engineers and teachers. Health care planning is necessary in order to match needs, demands and available resources within this complex system.

Resources

These can be considered under three headings:
financial;
manpower;
facilities.

Financial

The cost of modern medicine is now such that few people can afford to budget for it out of their income. In most countries where a state system of care does not exist, people insure themselves against medical expenses. The difficulty about this is that the risks of long-term illnesses are difficult for a commercial company to underwrite. Even if this were possible, high premiums would have to be imposed. The prevalence of chronic ill health increases with age and affects the individual's earning capacity. Thus the most vulnerable members of the community are the least able to maintain payment of premiums. This broadly describes the situation in the USA where further problems arise because the system has historically lacked means to limit both the level of professional fees and the number of treatments (operations and prescriptions, etc.) carried out. Health care costs in the USA are amongst the highest in the world, whereas large sections of the population, including especially the poor and the elderly, suffer medical neglect.

In order to overcome some of the obvious dangers of making each individual responsible for his or her own medical care, many countries have introduced state health care systems. These provide for the state either to underwrite high risk individuals or to offer state supervized and subsidized insurance. In all of these the state bears all or part of the cost from general taxation. In most such systems the user of services pays all or part of the cost and then reclaims a proportion from the insurance fund. This is said to be advantageous because it makes people aware of the true cost of medical care. This type of system operates in most western European countries other than the UK.

At the other extreme from the US system is the system operating in the Soviet Union and other Eastern European countries, where health services are entirely and directly State provided and funded and all staff are directly employed by the state. Such systems tend to be under funded, spending smaller percentages of a smaller national income on health services than Western societies. For example, the proportion of GNP spent on health in the Soviet Union is 3.5% compared with 5.5% in the UK, 10% in France and 11.5% in the USA.

The British system is unique in being funded from a combination of direct taxation and national insurance contributions to which are added a range of charges including prescription and dental charges, etc. Medical and other professional practitioners retain a large measure of professional independence, and responsible use of the service by the public is encouraged by the various charges made to patients.

Whatever the source of finance, there is a limit to the amount of money that individuals, governments or insurance companies will spend on health. It follows that if a high proportion of the available money is spent on one type of service, e.g. acute services, less is available for other important aspects of care, e.g. the care of the chronic sick. In a state system decisions about how the available money should be spent are political, and they must remain so, because the politicians carry the final responsibility for all public expenditure. In privately financed systems the balance is determined by the amount of money each individual has and is willing to spend. As the working, fit population have the greatest spending power this usually results in a growth of acute services to the detriment of chronic services.

Manpower

The second constraint on health service planning is the numbers and types of trained personnel that are available. The principal groups involved are doctors, nurses and technicians.

Absolute manpower deficiencies arise from a shortfall in national training programmmes, by net emigration of personnel, or by a sudden need to increase the staff available, such as may be caused by a change in therapy. In developed world absolute deficiencies are uncommon; manpower problems result from poor distribution. This will occur in two ways:

• Certain specialties may be less attractive to a young graduate than others. For example, it has always been easier to recruit general surgeons and physicians than it has been to attract people to geriatrics and psychiatry. Usually people tend to train for specialties that interest them rather than for those that are most needed.

• Some areas of the country are more desirable to live in than others; because of this there may be an over provision in some districts and severe deficit in others.

Equipment

The availability of sophisticated equipment can restrict the development of services even if manpower and finance is adequate. This is particularly important for planning new technological developments.

Needs

There is no absolute definition of 'need' for medical care. It is determined in part by the nature of the patients' problem and in part by what medical services can offer. Some needs are perceived by individuals for themselves. Other needs are not perceived by individuals but may be recognized by others (Fig. 17.1)

Perceived needs

Not all people who feel unwell seek professional assistance. They take action themselves, e.g. by going to bed for two days because of influenza or take advice

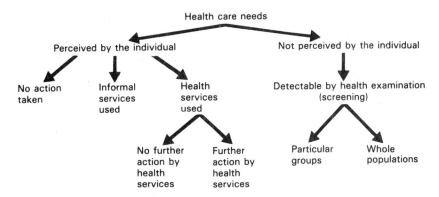

Fig. 17.1 Health care needs and the use of services.

from a friend or relative. Once they decide that they require medical intervention they make a demand on the health service. The doctor who sees the patient may or may not then accept that the problem will benefit from his skills. The only type of 'need' that can be measured without special study is that which creates a demand on the service.

Unperceived needs

An individual who is aware of his need for medical intervention has symptoms or signs which he associates with illness. However, the professional worker may detect signs of illness that is amenable to treatment in the absence of such symptoms. This requires screening or health examination surveys.

Demands

The work load of a health service is affected by the incidence of acute diseases (which are usually of short duration) and the prevalence of chronic diseases (for which care may be required over a long period of time). Demand is measured either by monitoring the workload of the service or by special surveys conducted in the population. Demands on services are not always an accurate method of measuring need. They are affected by:

knowledge of the existence of services;

local availability of services;

sectional pressure for intervention.

Knowledge of the existence of services

Without knowledge of the existence of a facility, e.g. total hip replacement, an individual will not make a demand for that service. He may, therefore, perceive a need to have his pain relieved, yet take no action. The publicity given to a particular service, e.g. by a television documentary, inevitably increases the perceived need and therefore increases demand.

Local availability of services

In some localities a particular service may not exist, or its availability may be so restricted that the individual does not trouble to try to use it. An example of this is the provision of long-stay geriatric accommodation, which may be so limited that many people make no effort to use the system.

Sectional pressure for intervention

Sectional pressure may create a demand for a service with limited relevance and sometimes questionable value to the community.

Unmet demand

The most obvious indication of unmet demand is a 'waiting list', which may be for an out-patient consultation, admission to hospital or even for a general practice consultation. For the reasons given below these are of limited value in service planning.

Interpretation of workload statistics

General practice

These consultations are usually initiated by the patient. These numbers will be affected by the user's perception of how available the doctor is, and of how relevant the doctor's skills are to his particular problem.

New out-patient referrals

These are initiated by a doctor (usually a GP). His interpretation of the patient's need for specialist advice or treatment and his assessment of his own skills, as well as the local availability of services, will affect the numbers of patients he refers.

Re-attendance

Re-attendance at out-patient clinics is also doctor-initiated, in this case by the doctor who is based within the clinic. The interpretation of such statistics is even more complex than in the case of new referrals. Typically when consultant retires the number of re-attendances at out-patients goes down because his successor tends to be more selective about who sees on a long-term basis.

Waiting lists for admissions

These are not always indicative of unmet demand, or of deficiencies, in the service. They are often necessary for the efficient functioning of a hospital. Without a modest waiting list it is not possible to ensure that hospital beds are used to capacity and it is expensive to leave them empty. A waiting list cannot be evaluated without taking account of the number of beds available and the expected length of stay of each patient. From these additional data it is possible to calculate the expected waiting time.

Waiting lists are also related to variables such as shortage of manpower, operating theatre time or equipment which may interfere with the normal flow of patients. Other factors include the personal reputation of individual consultants and the definition of and adherence to catchment areas. All of these should be taken into account when interpreting such statistics.

Bed occupancy

Several extremely useful indices of hospital bed utilization are published. These include the average number of beds occupied daily for different age/sex groups and the discharge rates for age/sex and disease groupings. All these indices are published on a national and regional basis.

Admission rates and lengths of stay vary with age. A large proportion of hospital beds are occupied by persons over the age of 65 because they have a high admission rate and tend to stay for long periods.

Formulating plans

Planning health services is a complex exercise. It takes place within a framework laid down by governments, who make general decisions on policies and finance.

Local plans should take account of the best possible estimates of local needs, both met and unmet. This generally requires using data relating to demand. In some circumstances, where such data may give a very distorted picture of real need, special surveys may have to be instituted. Some attempt should also be made to predict new needs and new demands. These estimates must then be applied to the projected population, taking account of its age and sex structure.

National Health Service (new arrangements)

The problem of matching the necessary finite resources which any society is able or willing to devote to health care to the potentially infinite demand for health care fuelled by rising public expectations, combined with the apparently limitless growth of medical technology is universal. It has led, in the UK during the 80s to a series of apparent financial crises in the NHS which have caused considerable public and governmental anxiety. In an attempt to improve the management and especially the financial efficiency of the service, a series of managerial reorganizations have been imposed culminating with what the government itself described as proposals for the most far reaching set of changes which NHS has undergone since its inception.

The proposed next reorganization seeks to introduce the disciplines of the market place into the NHS. It is to be achieved by separating the function of providing health services from that of paying for them. It is intended that DHAs and some General Practices should act as proxies for patients in purchasing hospital services. The hospitals will compete with each other to obtain treatment contracts from the purchasing authorities. In this way it is envisaged that the services providers will be stimulated to offering more efficient, cheaper and better quality services from which patients will benefit.

The current proposals are the subject of intense political controversy both as to the likelihood or otherwise of their achieving their declared purpose and as to the speed with which they are being implemented. Opponents of the proposals fear that financial constraints will override all other considerations leading to services being provided on price rather than quality and accessibility. It is also feared that financially unsuccessful hospitals will be forced into closure and that costly but 'unprofitable' services, such as those for the elderly, the chronically ill and the physically and mentally handicapped, will be uneconomic and thus will not be provided. Against this pessimism it is argued that the organization of health services in many of the EEC countries bears a close resemblance to that being proposed by the government. Most of those countries have managed to provide a truly comprehensive health care system of high quality. They have also managed to combine publicly financed provision with freedom of choice. However, none has been able to contain the rising costs of medical care.

Appendix
Suggested Further Reading

Acheson R M, Hagard S. *Health, Society and Medicine: An Introduction to Community Medicine*. Oxford: Blackwell Scientific Publications, 1984.

Armitage P, Berry G. *Statistical Methods in Medical Research*. Oxford: Blackwell Scientific Publications, 1987.

Armstrong D. *An Outline of Sociology as Applied to Medicine*. 3rd edn. Bristol: John Wright, 1989.

Barker D J P, Rose G. *Epidemiology in Medical Practice*. 4th edn. Edinburgh: Churchill Livingstone, 1990.

Black N, Boswell D, Gray A, Murphy S, Popay J. *Health and Diseases: A Reader*. Milton Keynes: Open University Press, 1984.

Bland M. *An Introduction to Medical Statistics*. Oxford: Oxford University Press, 1987.

Chaplin N W, (ed.) *Health Care in the United Kingdom: Its Organisation and Management*. London: Kluwer Medical, 1982.

Cochrane A L. *Effectiveness and Efficiency: Random Reflections in Health Services*. London: British Medical Association and Nuffield Provincial Hospital Trust, reprinted 1989.

Donaldson R J, Donaldson L J. *Essential Community Medicine*. Lancester: MTP Press, 1983.

Emond R T D, Bradley J M, Galbraith N S. *Infection*. 2nd edn. Oxford: Blackwell Scientific Publications, 1989.

Joint Committee on Vaccination & Immunisation. *Immunisation Against Infectious Diseases*. London: HMSO, 1990.

Levitt R, Wall A. *The Reorganised National Health Service*. 3rd edn. London: Croom Helm, 1984.

Lilienfield A M, Lilienfield D. *Foundations of Epidemiology*. 2nd edn. Oxford: Oxford University Press, 1980.

McKeown T. *The Role of Medicine*. Oxford: Basil Blackwell, 1980.

Miller D L, Farmer R D T. *Epidemiology of Diseases*. Oxford: Blackwell Scientific Publications, 1982.

Patrick D L, Scambler G. (eds.) *Sociology as Applied to Medicine*. 2nd edn. London: Bailliere Tindall, 1986.

Richards I D G, Baker M R. *Epidemiology and Prevention of Important Diseases*. London: Churchill Livingstone, 1988.

Smith A, Jacobson B. (eds.) *The Nations Health: A Strategy for the 1990s*. London: King Edward's Hospital Fund for London, 1988.

Townsend P, Davidson N. *Inequalities in Health (The Black Report)*. London: Penguin Books, 1982.

Waldron H A. *Lecture Notes on Occupational Medicine*. 4th edn. Oxford: Blackwell Scientific Publications, 1990.

Index

Italics refer to pages with figures and/or tables.